Rethinking School Feeding: Social
Safety Nets, Child Development,
and the Education Sector

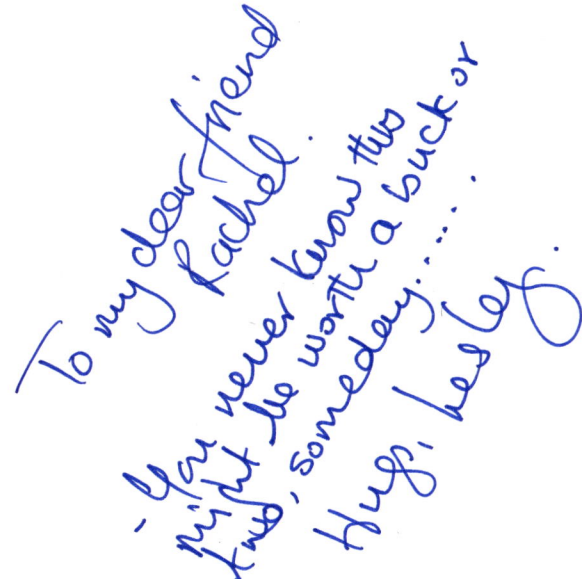

To my dear friend
Rachel.
- You never know this
might be worth a buck or
two, someday......
Hugs, Lesley

# Rethinking School Feeding: Social Safety Nets, Child Development, and the Education Sector

*Authors*
Donald Bundy
Carmen Burbano
Margaret Grosh
Aulo Gelli
Matthew Jukes
Lesley Drake

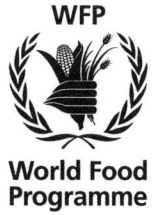

**WFP**

**World Food Programme**

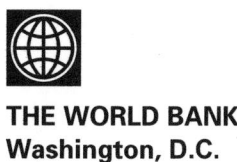

**THE WORLD BANK**
**Washington, D.C.**

1818 H Street NW
Washington DC 20433
Telephone: 202-473-1000
Internet: www.worldbank.org
E-mail: feedback@worldbank.org

ISBN: 978-0-8213-7974-5
eISBN: 978-0-8213-7975-2
DOI: 10.1596/978-0-8213-7974-5

**Library of Congress Cataloging-in-Publication Data**

Rethinking school feeding : social safety nets, child development, and the education sector /  by Donald Bundy ... [et al.].
     p. cm. — (Directions in development)
     Includes bibliographical references and index.
     ISBN 978-0-8213-7974-5 (alk. paper) — ISBN 978-0-8213-7975-2 (electronic)
     1. School children—Food. 2. Children—Nutrition. I. Bundy, Donald A. P.

     LB3475.R48 2009
     371.7'16—dc22

                                                                                    2009017125

Cover photo by: Marcus Prior, World Food Programme.
Cover design by: Naylor Design, Inc.

# Contents

## Boxes

## Figures

**Maps**

**Tables**

# Foreword

The year 2009 will be a dangerous one. Before the financial crisis hit last year, soaring food and fuel prices pushed 130 to 155 million people into extreme poverty. This year, because of the financial crisis, the World Bank Group estimates that there will be 53 million more people living in extreme poverty. As is always the case, the poorest are the most vulnerable, especially children. According to the UN World Food Programme, in developing countries almost 60 million children go to school hungry every day—about 40 percent of them are in Africa. The prospect of reaching the UN's Millennium Development Goals by 2015, already a cause for serious concern, now looks even more distant.

In the poorest countries, school feeding programs are emerging as a common social safety net response to crisis. In 2008, 20 governments looked to school feeding programs as a safety net response to protect the poorest. The UN World Food Programme assisted some 22 million children with school feeding in 70 countries, and the World Bank Group launched a Global Food Crisis Response Facility that mobilized $1.2 billion to help countries respond to the food and fuel crises, including by scaling-up school feeding programs.

School feeding programs provide an important new opportunity to assist poor families and feed hungry children. These programs have the potential to combat hunger and support nutrition through micronutrient-fortified food and deworming. They can provide an incentive for poor families to send their children to school—and keep them there—while improving their children's education. And these programs can be targeted to benefit the most vulnerable, especially girls and children affected by Human Immunodeficiency Virus (HIV). These potential benefits come with potential costs, however, particularly in terms of opportunities foregone, an increased burden on the education sector, and the fiscal challenge of long-term commitment.

This joint publication of the World Food Programme and the World Bank Group, *Rethinking School Feeding: Social Safety Nets, Child Development, and the Education Sector*, provides a new analysis of school feeding programs. It benefits from combining the World Food Programme's practical experience in running school feeding programs with the World Bank Group's development policy dialogue and analysis. It explores how food procurement may help local economies and emphasizes the centrality of the education sector in the policy dialogue on school feeding. This study can help governments, policy makers, donors, nongovernmental organizations, and other partners to explore the costs and benefits of school feeding programs. It can also help them circumnavigate the pitfalls and trade-offs in designing effective programs that are capable of responding quickly to today's crises, while maintaining fiscally sustainable investments in children's education and general human potential in the long term.

A key message from this paper is that the transition to sustainable national programs depends on mainstreaming school feeding into national policies and plans, especially education sector plans. What is also clear from this report is that we are beyond the debate about whether school feeding makes sense as a way to reach the most vulnerable. It does. In the face of global crises, we must now focus on how school feeding programs can be designed and implemented in a cost-effective and sustainable way to benefit and protect those most in need of help today and in the future.

*Josette Sheeran*
Executive Director
World Food Programme

*Robert Zoellick*
President
The World Bank Group

# Acknowledgments

This document was written by Donald Bundy (World Bank), Carmen Burbano (World Food Programme), Margaret Grosh (World Bank), Aulo Gelli (Imperial College), Matthew Jukes (Harvard University), and Lesley Drake (Partnership for Child Development). Guidance for its preparation was led by the Chief Economist of the Human Development Network of the World Bank, Ariel Fiszbein; and the Chief of School Feeding Policy of the World Food Programme, Nancy Walters.

The peer reviewers for the document were Harold Alderman and Emiliana Vegas, from the World Bank, and Ute Meir and Steven Were Omamo, from the World Food Programme.

We would like to thank the following people for their direct contributions to this document: Deborah Hines (World Food Programme [WFP]) gave input on the sustainability of school feeding and coordinated the drafting of the case studies; Kristie Neeser (Partnership for Child Development [PCD]) contributed with preparation of the maps, case studies, tables, and appendixes; Emilio Porta (World Bank [WB]), Federica Carfagna (WFP), Fahma Nur (WB), and Felipe Barrera (WB) contributed to the maps; and Claire Risley (PCD) developed figures 4.1 and 4.2 in chapter 4. Additional inputs, especially for the case studies, were provided by Luis Benveniste, Samuel Carlson, Peter Holland, Carlo del Ninno, and David Warren from the World Bank; Ana Garcia, Agnes Mallipu, Daysi Marquez, Rene McGuffin, Margarita Sanchez, Carlo Scaramella, and Adrian Storbeck from WFP; and Rachel Winch from the Global Child Nutrition Foundation. Editorial support was provided by Anastasia Said (PCD).

We gratefully acknowledge the technical feedback from the following people: from the World Bank—Colin Andrews, Simeth Beng, Raja Bentaouet, Luis Benveniste, Lynn Brown, Helen Craig, Amit Dar, Peter Holland, Stella Manda, Menno Mulder-Sibanda, Claudia Rokx, Ludovic Subran, Jee-Peng Tan, Andy Chi Tembon, Christopher Thomas, Alexandria Valerio, and Eduardo Velez; from the World Food Programme—Abdallah Alwardat, John Aylieff, Bill Barclay, Cora Best, Rita Bhatia, Alphonsine Bouya, Tina van den Briel, Federica Carfagna, Jose Castillo, Claudio Delicato, Francisco Espejo, Catherine Feeney, Ugo Gentilini, Salha Hamdani, Edith Heines, Paul Howe, Allan Jury, Joyce Luma, Agnes Mallipu, Karin Manente, Jakob Mikkelsen, Leo Nederveen, Mary Njoroge, Marc Regnault de la Mothe, Janne Suvanto, Paul Turnbull, and Hildegard Tuttinghoff; Koli Banik and Robert Prouty from the Education for All-Fast Track Initiative Secretariat; Arlene Mitchell from the Bill & Melinda Gates Foundation; and Daniel Gilligan from the International Food Policy Research Institute.

Finally, we would also like to thank all those who participated in the World Bank Learning Week event in November 2008 and the World Food Programme School Feeding Strategy meeting in December 2008, whose contributions helped shape the conclusions of this document.

# Abbreviations

| | |
|---|---|
| AIDS | Acquired Immune Deficiency Syndrome |
| APR | Annual Performance Report |
| BMI | body mass index |
| CAR | Central African Republic |
| CCT | conditional cash transfer |
| CRS | Catholic Relief Services |
| DRC | Democratic Republic of Congo |
| EFA | Education for All |
| FAO | Food and Agriculture Organization of the United Nations |
| FCI | Food Corporation of India |
| FNDE | National Fund for the Development of Education (in Brazil) |
| FRESH | Focusing Resources on Effective School Health |
| FTI | Fast Track Initiative |
| g | gram |
| GDP | gross domestic product |
| HGSF | home-grown school feeding |
| HIV | Human Immunodeficiency Virus |
| IDA | iron deficiency anemia |
| IFPRI | International Food Policy Research Institute |

| | |
|---|---|
| kcal | kilocalorie |
| kg | kilogram |
| Kshs | Kenya shillings |
| M&E | monitoring and evaluation |
| MDG | Millennium Development Goal |
| MDM | Mid-Day Meals |
| MNP | micronutrient powder |
| NEPAD | New Partnership for Africa's Development |
| NGO | nongovernmental organization |
| OECD | Organisation for Economic Co-operation and Development |
| OVC | orphans and vulnerable children |
| PCD | Partnership for Child Development |
| PNCS | National School Feeding Program (in Haiti) |
| PRSP | Poverty Reduction Strategy Paper |
| SD | standard deviation |
| SEAMEO | Southeast Asian Ministers of Education Organization |
| SMC | School Management Committee |
| SPR | Standard Project Report |
| UNESCO | United Nations Educational, Scientific and Cultural Organization |
| UNICEF | United Nations Children's Fund |
| US | United States |
| USAID | U.S. Agency for International Development |
| VAM | Vulnerability Analysis and Mapping |
| WB | World Bank |
| WFP | World Food Programme |
| WHO | World Health Organization |

# Executive Summary

This review was undertaken jointly by the World Food Programme (WFP) and the World Bank Group, building on the comparative advantages of both organizations. The overall objective is to provide guidance on how to develop and implement effective school feeding programs, in the context of both a productive safety net, as part of the response to the social shocks of the current global crises, as well as a fiscally sustainable investment in human capital as part of long-term global efforts to achieve Education for All and provide social protection for the poor.

The analysis was initiated in response to enhanced demand for school feeding programs from low-income countries affected by the social shocks of the current global crises, and focused first on the role of school feeding as a social safety net. This proved to be too narrow a context, and the analyses evolved to address the longer-term implications for social protection and the development of human capital as part of national policy.

This shift in emphasis came about because the available data suggest that today, perhaps for the first time in history, every country for which we have information is seeking to provide food, in some way and at some scale, to its schoolchildren. The coverage is most complete in the rich and middle-income countries—indeed, it seems that most countries that can afford to provide food for their schoolchildren do so. But where the need is greatest—in terms of hunger, poverty, and poor social indicators—the programs tend to be the smallest, though usually targeted to the most food-insecure regions. These programs are also those most reliant on external support, and nearly all are supported by WFP.

So the key issue today is not whether countries will implement school feeding programs, but how and with what objective. The near universality of school feeding provides important opportunities for WFP, the World Bank, and other development partners to assist governments in rolling out productive safety nets as part of the response to the current global crises, and also to sow the seeds for school feeding programs to grow into fiscally sustainable investments in human capital.

## The Benefits of School Feeding Programs

School feeding programs provide an explicit or implicit transfer to households of the value of the food distributed. The programs are relatively easy to scale up in a crisis and can provide a benefit per household of more than 10 percent of household expenditures, even more in the case of take-home rations. In many contexts, well-designed school feeding programs can be targeted moderately accurately, though rarely so effectively as the most progressive of cash transfers. In the poorest countries, where school enrollment is low, school feeding may not reach the poorest people, but in these settings alternative safety net options are often quite limited, and geographically targeted expansion of school feeding may still provide the best option for rapid scale-up of safety nets. Targeted take-home rations may provide somewhat more progressive outcomes. Further research is required to assess the longer-term relative merits of school feeding versus other social safety net instruments in these situations.

There is evidence that school feeding programs increase school attendance, cognition, and educational achievement, particularly if supported by complementary actions such as deworming and micronutrient fortification or supplementation. In many cases the programs have a strong gender dimension, especially where they target girls' education, and may also be used to benefit specifically the poorest and most vulnerable children. What is less clear is the relative scale of the benefit with the different school feeding modalities, and there is a notable lack of engagement of educators on research around these issues.

The clear education benefits of the programs are a strong justification for the education sector to own and implement the programs, while these same education outcomes contribute to the incentive compatibility of the programs for social protection. Policy analysis also shows that the effectiveness and sustainability of school feeding programs is dependent upon embedding the programs within education sector policy. Hence, the value of school feeding as a safety net and the motivation of the education sector to implement the programs are both enhanced by the extent to which there are education benefits.

Well-designed school feeding programs, which include micronutrient fortification and deworming, can provide nutritional benefits and should complement and not compete with nutrition programs for younger children, which remain a clear priority for targeting malnutrition overall.

## The Sustainability of School Feeding Programs

The concept of a school feeding "exit strategy" has tended to confound thinking about the longer-term future of school feeding programs. Here we show that countries do not seek to exit from providing food to their schoolchildren, but rather to transition from externally supported projects to national programs. For 28 countries previously assisted by WFP, this has already happened, and here we begin to review case studies of how externally assisted programs transition into sustainable national programs, which in some cases have themselves gone on to provide technical support to others (for example, Brazil, Chile, and India).

This review highlights three main findings. First, school feeding programs in low-income countries exhibit large variation in cost, with concomitant opportunities for cost containment. Second, as countries get richer, school feeding costs become a much smaller proportion of the investment in education. For example, in Zambia the cost of school feeding is about 50 percent of annual per capita costs for primary education; in Ireland it is only 10 percent. Further analysis is required to define these relationships, but supporting countries to maintain an investment in school feeding through this transition may emerge as a key role for development partners. Third, the main preconditions for the transition to sustainable national programs are mainstreaming school feeding in national policies and plans, especially education sector plans; identifying national sources of financing; and expanding national implementation capacity. Mainstreaming a development policy for school feeding into national education sector plans offers the added advantage of aligning support for school feeding with the processes already established to harmonize development partner support for the Education for All-Fast Track Initiative.

A key message is the importance of both designing long-term sustainability into programs from their inception and of revisiting programs as they evolve. Countries benefit from having a clear understanding of the duration of donor assistance, a systematic strategy to strengthen institutional capacity, and a concrete plan for the transition to national ownership with time frames and milestones for the process.

## Trade-Offs in the Design of School Feeding Programs

The effectiveness of school feeding programs is dependent upon several factors, including the selection of modality (in-school meals, fortified biscuits, take-home rations, or some combination of these); the effectiveness of targeting; and the associated costs.

Take-home rations (average per capita cost US$50 per year) can be more finely targeted and can give high-value transfers, but have significant administrative costs. They have strong safety net potential and appear to result in increases in attendance, and perhaps educational achievement, on a similar scale to in-school meal programs. Thus, from a social protection point of view they may be preferred to in-school meal programs.

In-school meals (average per capita cost US$40 per year) tend to be less finely targeted and capped in the value of their transfer, have potentially large opportunity costs for education, and incur higher administrative costs, but have the potential not only to increase attendance but to act more directly on learning, especially if fortified and combined with deworming. In-school snacks and biscuits (average per capita cost US$13 per year) have lower administrative costs but also lower transfer and incentive value, though the scale of benefit relative to meals needs to be better quantified.

Designing effective programs that meet their objectives requires an evidence base that allows careful trade-offs among targeting approaches, feeding modalities, and costs. There is a particular need for better data on the cost-effectiveness of the available approaches and modalities. There are very few studies that compare in-school feeding with take-home rations in similar settings, and the few that have gone further with this suggest that both programs lead to similar improvements over having no program at all.

The key issue is that in selecting any modality, there are important trade-offs dependent upon context, benefit, and cost. In some contexts, for example, school feeding programs combine on-site meals with an extra incentive from take-home rations targeting a specific group of vulnerable children, such as those affected by HIV or girls in higher grades.

## Institutional and Procurement Arrangements

The appropriate approach to implementing school feeding programs will vary depending on the program objectives; the context, that is, whether the program is implemented in stable, conflict, or emergency situations; the capacity of the government at different levels to manage the program using its staff, infrastructure, and accountability systems; the type of resources available from local and external sources, whether cash or in-kind; and the presence of key implementing partners, especially those organizations specializing in school feeding programs.

Case studies of programs that have transitioned to national ownership show that effective programs have a designated national institution, usually the education sector, and well-developed capacity at the subnational levels. While national ownership appears to be a critical factor, many different approaches to implementation—including public sector, private sector, and public-private partnerships—appear to be effective.

The management of school feeding programs has become increasingly decentralized, mirroring the trend in the education sector toward school-based management. But the extent of involvement of teachers and education staff is an important issue because there are, for example, very significant opportunity costs of using teachers to prepare food.

The design of school feeding programs should specifically address the following significant issues and challenges: environmental concerns related to cooking fuel and disposal of commodity packaging; inappropriate use of school gardens for food production; and the potential opportunities for corrupt practices in procurement and contracting.

The roles and responsibilities of the institutional system depend largely on the procurement modality and sources of food: local procurement is the most common approach within national programs and is emerging as the more common approach overall. Local procurement is being actively evaluated as a means to achieve sustainable school feeding programs and, at the same time, to use the purchasing power of the program as a stimulus for the local agricultural economy. As such, local purchase of food for school feeding is seen as a force multiplier, benefiting children and the local economy at the same time.

## Toolkits to Design and Update School Feeding Programs

An important conclusion of these analyses is that there is a need to improve the initial design of school feeding programs and, where necessary, to update existing programs. To support these processes, the book presents two new tools, one to facilitate the initial design of school feeding programs, and the other to help update existing programs. These checklists are complemented by an array of design and assessment tools.

This review also proposes a research agenda to fill in some important gaps in current knowledge, with the aim of creating a stronger evidence base for future decision making.

## The Way Forward

The overall conclusion is that the global food, fuel, and financial crises and the refocusing of government efforts on school feeding that has followed, provide an important new opportunity to help children today and to revisit national policies and planning for long-term sustainability tomorrow. Taking full advantage of this opportunity will require a more systematic and policy-driven approach to school feeding by both governments and development partners.

# CHAPTER 1

# Context and Rationale

This review was undertaken jointly by the World Food Programme (WFP) and the World Bank, building on the comparative advantages of both organizations. This partnership was strengthened to address the school feeding responses precipitated by the global food crisis, but has evolved to address the fiscal sustainability of productive safety nets in response to the long-term objectives of countries.

The overall objective is to provide guidance on how to develop and implement effective school feeding programs, in the context of both a productive safety net as part of the response to the social shocks of the current global crises, and a fiscally sustainable investment in human capital as part of long-term global efforts to achieve Education for All (EFA) and provide social protection for the poor. The review is targeted at the education and social protection sectors, but may also be relevant to the health sector in countries where school health and school feeding are coordinated by the health sector. The review seeks to provide an analysis of the evidence for benefits from school feeding programs and to offer evidence-based guidance on the design and operation of school feeding programs. To the extent possible, this review uses recent published and unpublished sources to develop an evidence base and builds on earlier literature, especially on the role of school feeding in the education sector.

The global food, fuel, and financial crises have given new prominence to school feeding as a potential safety net and as a social support measure that helps keep children in school. Evidence from previous real income shocks suggests that there is a significant risk to educational outcomes for the poor as a result of increases in commodity prices. The 1997 economic crisis in Indonesia was associated with a doubling of the numbers of out-of-school children (Frankenberg et al. 1999), while droughts in Sub-Saharan Africa have been associated with declines in both schooling and child nutrition (Schady 2008). In the current crisis, about half the households surveyed in Bangladesh had reduced spending on education to cope with rising food prices, with girls particularly at risk (Grosh, del Ninno, and Tesliuc 2008).

But good safety net programs take time to develop and in crises the emphasis in the short run is on scaling up existing programs. In many settings, school feeding is potentially the largest and often the only direct transfer program that can be used for a quick response. Expanding existing school feeding programs can provide a point of entry to the community: they are politically popular, they exist in many countries, and where there is an insufficient cash transfer program, school feeding can be a starting point for a rapid response. Conversely, disruption of existing school feeding programs has almost immediate negative social consequences, especially for girls, removing children from the school environment and enhancing vulnerability. Because of the value of school feeding as a social safety net and as a measure to mitigate impacts on education, the World Bank Group specifically included school feeding as eligible for support from the US$1.2 billion Global Food Crisis Response Facility established in fiscal year 2008 (Grosh, del Ninno, and Tesliuc 2008).

To assess the relevance of current school feeding programs in this expanded role, we compare the current provision of school feeding programs globally with current estimates of the global patterns of hunger, poverty, and underachievement in education (see maps 1.1 through 1.4). This is a first attempt at a global school feeding map, and should be viewed as a work in progress. Indeed, all the maps should be interpreted cautiously because they describe an average situation for each country, which may mask important underlying regional differences. With these caveats in mind, three conclusions are apparent. First, the countries with the greatest need are those where the school feeding programs are currently least adequate. Second, comprehensive school feeding is near universal in those high- and middle-income countries that can afford the programs and for which data are available. Third, it appears that every country for which we have data is in some way and at some scale seeking to provide food to its schoolchildren.

The ubiquity of school feeding programs suggests that these programs are indeed appropriate candidates for a rapid safety net response. But it also testifies to the popularity of these programs and reinforces the perception that an increasing number of governments have the policy intention of establishing school feeding as a long-term intervention. This has at least two important policy implications. First, it addresses the concern that reaction to the current crisis may saddle governments with school feeding programs that may be unwanted once the crisis is over, but difficult to terminate for political reasons. The current observations suggest instead that such programs are already in place in most countries, and that the priority, therefore, is to support government efforts to ensure that these programs are meaningfully integrated into national development policies and plans where there is government demand. Second, and as a natural consequence of the first implication, there is a need for program design to address the issue of long-term sustainability from the outset, because for many countries it appears that the political vision is for the short-term response to have the inbuilt ability to translate into a sustainable human capital investment program in the longer term. However, analysis elsewhere in this book suggests that the process of scaling up programs benefits from a clear expression by governments of their national long-term policy and support for school feeding in the context of a national development strategy.

The renewed focus on school feeding in the context of education and safety nets has resulted in demand for up-to-date sectoral guidance on the key issues in developing school feeding programs. Early experience with the expansion of school feeding programs under the World Bank Group's 2008 response to the food price crisis shows that while the overall project is often prepared by the agriculture or social protection sectors, the school feeding subcomponent is typically prepared by the education sector team. This review aims to provide an evidence-based rationale for school feeding from a social protection and education perspective and provide operational guidance on the design and implementation of school feeding programs.

**Map 1.1    Poverty: Percentage of Population Living in Households with Consumption or Income per Person below the Poverty Line**

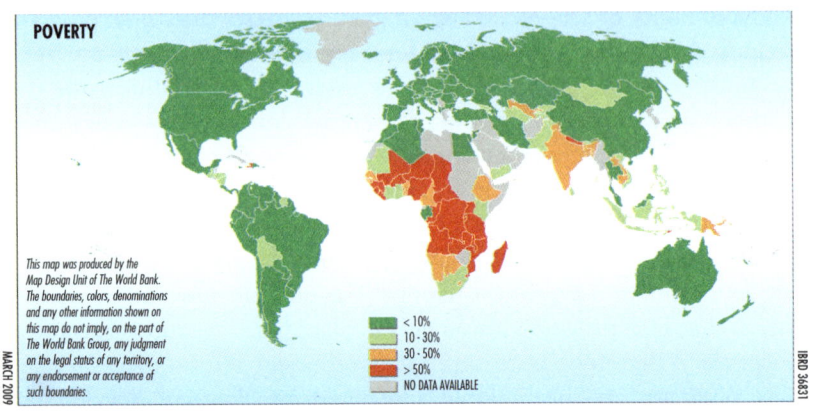

*Source:* World Bank 2008.
*Note:* The poverty line estimates use Purchasing Power Parity exchange rates for latest available year.

**Map 1.2    Hunger: Percentage of Population below the Minimum Level of Dietary Energy Consumption, 2002–05**

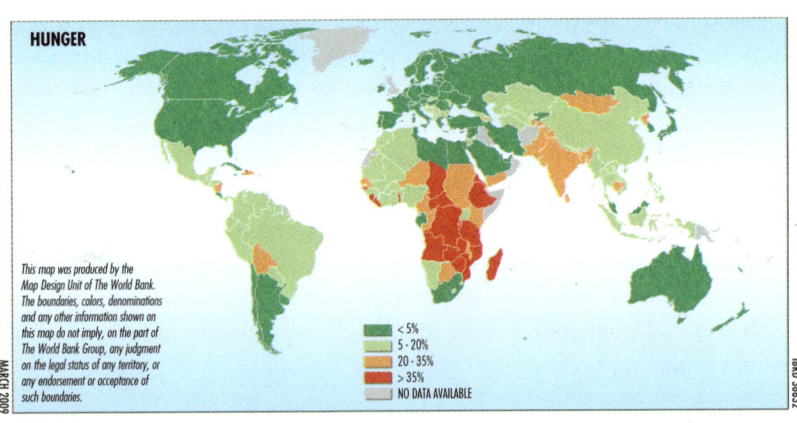

*Source:* FAO 2007, 2008.
*Note:* The proportion of the population below the minimum level of dietary energy consumption, referred to as the prevalence of undernourishment, is the percentage of the population that is undernourished or food deprived. Figures are from latest available year. Standards derived from an FAO/WHO/UNU Expert Consultation (FAO, WHO, and UN University 2004).

## Map 1.3    Primary School Completion Rate, Total, 2000–06

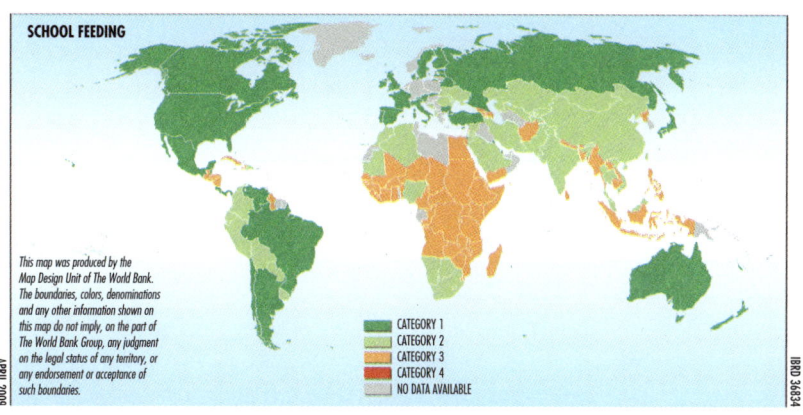

*Source:* UNESCO 2008.

*Note:* Primary completion rate is the total number of students in grade 6 (excluding repeaters) divided by the total number of children of grade age. Figures are from latest available year. All data are from the UNESCO Institute for Statistics except for Australia, Canada, China, Japan, New Zealand, Sweden, Thailand, and the United Kingdom, which are from national data.

## Map 1.4    School Feeding: Country Programs, 2006–08

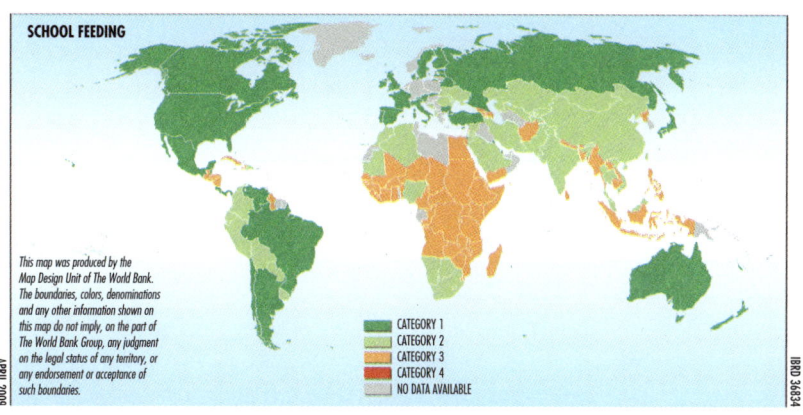

*Source:* http://www.schoolsandhealth.org/Pages/SchoolNutritionFoodforEducation.aspx.

*Note:* Category 1: Countries where school feeding is available in most schools, sometimes or always; Category 2: Countries where school feeding is available in some way and at some scale; Category 3: Countries where school feeding is available primarily in the most food-insecure regions; Category 4: Countries where there is no school feeding. The sources, as detailed in the database link, are WFP data for low-income and lower-middle-income countries and national data for the remaining countries. Because this is a work in progress, comments and any further information on school feeding programs are welcomed.

# CHAPTER 2

# What Is School Feeding?

School feeding programs use many different modalities to provide food to schoolchildren. There are also complementary actions that, at marginal cost and implemented as part of the program, can add to the effectiveness of school feeding programs. In addition, there are important larger contexts that affect the efficiency and outcomes of school feeding and should be included in the overall planning process. This chapter describes the main components of school feeding programs and some complementary actions, as well as explains the different program modalities and their terminology.

## The Food

School feeding is defined here as the provision of food to schoolchildren. There are as many types of programs as there are countries, but they can be classified into two main groups based on their modalities: in-school feeding, where children are fed in school; and take-home rations, where families are given food if their children attend school. In-school feeding can, in turn, be divided into two common categories: programs that provide meals, and programs that provide high-energy biscuits or snacks.

In some countries, in-school meals are combined with take-home rations for particularly vulnerable students, including girls and children affected by HIV, to generate greater impacts on school enrollment and retention rates, and reduce gender or social gaps.

### In-School Feeding

- *Meals.* For programs that provide meals, the primary objective is to provide breakfast, mid-morning meals, lunch, or a combination (depending on the duration of the school day) to alleviate short-term hunger, increase attention span, facilitate learning, and obviate the need for children to leave the school to find food. In-school meals also act as an incentive to increase school access. School meals can be prepared in schools or in the community, or can be delivered from centralized kitchens. They can be an important source of micronutrients if prepared using fortified commodities, or if micronutrient powder is added during or after preparation.

- *Fortified high-energy biscuits and snacks.* This program modality functions in a similar way to in-school meals, alleviating short-term hunger and micronutrient deficiencies, and improving learning. They can be part of a meals program, particularly in full-day schools, in which case they are given early in the day to alleviate short-term hunger. They are cheaper and easier to distribute than meals, and often aim to act as an incentive for increased school access, but they are less substantial and their financial value to families is lower. Biscuits are a compact source of nutrients produced off-site that is easy to pack, store, and transport. They are particularly used in emergency or crisis contexts for rapid scale-up or in situations of poor school infrastructure and storage facilities. Snacks require little preparation time and facilities, can be served early in the school day, and typically use fortified commodities such as blended foods. However, their use presumes the availability of safe drinking water because they are typically dry, and their nutritional content is lower than that of meals.

### Take-Home Rations

Take-home rations function in a similar manner to conditional cash transfers. They transfer food resources to families conditional upon school enrollment and regular attendance of children. Rations are given to families typically once a month or once a term. They increase school participation and probably learning. While they may require less school involvement than in-school modalities, they do demand an investment of school time in regular monitoring of the attendance condition. Their effect depends on whether the value of the ration offsets some of the costs of sending the child to school.

## Complementary Health and Nutrition Interventions

The addition of micronutrients to food (fortification), the delivery of micronutrients in pills or suspensions (supplementation), and the provision of anthelmintic treatment (deworming) are all cost-effective ways of enhancing the nutrition and education of schoolchildren.

These actions are viewed as complementary in the sense that food could be provided without these interventions, and because micronutrient supplements and deworming can be delivered independently of school feeding. There is a strong case, however, that micronutrient fortification should be an integral part of school feeding, and that deworming should be conducted alongside school feeding wherever there is an epidemiologically demonstrated need. This is now policy with World Food Programme (WFP) school feeding programs, in which case these may be viewed as essential actions.

### Micronutrient Fortification of Food and Micronutrient Supplementation

Micronutrient fortification is a low-cost means of including in meals or fortified biscuits or snacks the essential vitamins or minerals that may otherwise be deficient in the diet. The main micronutrients that are added are iron, iodine, vitamin A, B-vitamins, and zinc. Micronutrients can be added at the processing stage, as is the case with salt, oil, flour, and other foods. A new technology is the addition after the food has been cooked, using micronutrient powder. Fortification increases the intake of micronutrients, thereby improving micronutrient status, preventing damage caused by micronutrient deficiencies, and increasing cognition and nutritional status. School health and nutrition services may provide micronutrient supplements, most commonly iron supplements, in contexts where micronutrient deficiencies such as anemia are highly prevalent.

### Deworming

School-based deworming is a very low-cost and cost-effective way of improving education outcomes and nutrition. It involves offering deworming tablets once or twice a year to all children in schools in infection endemic areas. This delivery is readily incorporated into school feeding schedules. Reducing the prevalence and intensity of worm infections in children enhances nutritional status and learning and cognition, and reduces absenteeism. The greatest benefit is observed in the most vulnerable schoolchildren—the ones in lower grades, the most heavily infected, and the malnourished.

## Other Important Actions

It is perhaps worth recalling at this stage that the key purpose of schools is to provide education. There is an extensive literature on the many education interventions that are specifically intended to enhance student learning (see, for example, Vegas and Petrow [2007]) and these will not be discussed here. Instead, we focus on health interventions that offer the additional benefit of helping children learn.

There are health and nutrition interventions that help reinforce the benefits of school feeding programs and should be strongly promoted, but are typically part of broader sectoral and cross-sectoral policies and programs. The framework for Focusing Resources on Effective School Health (FRESH), launched at the World Education Forum in Dakar, Senegal, in 2000 by the United Nations Educational, Scientific, and Cultural Organization, the World Health Organization, the United Nations Children's Fund, the World Bank, WFP, and other partners, supports Education for All (Bundy et al. 2006). This framework specifically highlights the importance of implementing four elements together, in all schools: effective school health and nutrition policies; a safe and sanitary school environment with potable water; health, hygiene, and nutrition education; and school-based health and nutrition services, such as school feeding and deworming. WFP and UNICEF, along with other partners, support the implementation of an Essential Package of 12 complementary interventions, inspired by the Focusing Resources on Effective School Health (FRESH) framework, all of which provide for a supportive context for the delivery of school feeding and may reinforce the effects (WFP and UNICEF 2005).

Given that school feeding brings more children into school (see box 2.1), one particularly important issue to include in overall planning is to ensure that education provision is able to respond in quality and quantity to the increased education demand resulting from school feeding programs. This is a lesson learned by many countries through their experience of abolishing school fees and other financial barriers to education, and then having to respond to increased demand after the fact (Kattan 2006).

**Box 2.1**

## Case Studies: School Feeding Programs in Transition Stage 5
(for further details, see table 4.1)

### India

India has a long tradition of school feeding programs (some since the 1920s), largely funded by state governments with some external assistance. In 2001, India's Supreme Court directed state governments to introduce school feeding programs in all government and government-assisted primary schools. This was the result of a petition from the People's Union for Civil Liberties, a large coalition of organizations and individuals that led the Right to Food Campaign.

The Mid-Day Meal Program operates through the Food Corporation of India (FCI), which procures food domestically and then distributes it to a network of FCI stores, where it is then transported to individual schools and villages. The program is largely decentralized by the state, with operations varying throughout the country. The central government supports the states by providing free food grains (for example, rice or wheat) to implementing state agencies and reimbursing the costs of transportation to the district authorities. States pay for any additional food items required and for food preparation. States can choose from providing cooked meals at school or dry rations. Efforts have been made since 2001 to improve school infrastructure for the program, especially with the construction of kitchens, and to tackle challenges related to clean water, appropriate utensils, and eating facilities. Still, challenges remain in guaranteeing the quality and stability of the program in all states in the country under a decentralized system. Currently, the program has near universal coverage, reaching 130 million schoolchildren throughout India.

### Brazil

The Brazilian school feeding program is in the country's national constitution and is part of the government's Zero Hunger Program. Covering nearly 37 million children

*(continued)*

**Box 2.1** *(Continued)*

each year, the program is among the largest in the world. Its implementation is managed by an independent institution, the National Fund for Development of Education (FNDE), created in 1997 to be responsible for the disbursement of the financial resources for school meals in each municipality. This transfer became automatic in 2001 and obliges local governments to spend at least 70 percent of transferred money on food, preferably purchased locally.

The implementation modality in Brazil is highly decentralized. Regions, districts, and communities have a prominent role, not only in the day-to-day implementation of the program but also in decision-making processes. The role of FNDE is crucial to providing general guidance, standards, guidelines, audit and control systems, and efficient resource management. Food is bought through a tendering process, governed by law, that envisages an invitation process, pricing, public tendering, and a price registration system. The 1994 law obliges each municipal and state government to create a School Feeding Committee, representing different parts of the society, to be the local body and make fiscal arrangements for the school feeding program. This helps counter corruption. The School Feeding Committee also helps design a locally acceptable menu and promotes food procurement from local or regional sources. As of early 2009, Brazil was considering legislation to establish that at least 30 percent of the food used by the school feeding program should be procured locally (WFP 2009).

# CHAPTER 3

# Why Implement School Feeding?

There are three main reasons why countries may choose to implement school feeding programs: to address social needs and to provide a social safety net during crises; to improve learning and educational outcomes; and to enhance nutrition. The analyses below show that the evidence of benefit is particularly strong for safety nets and for education and that the responses in both of these sectors appear to contribute to gender equity.

## School Feeding as a Safety Net

School feeding programs are often used for social protection purposes as much as or more than for education goals. The programs provide an explicit or implicit transfer to households of the value of the food distributed, with the value of the transfer varying significantly from in-school snacks at the lower end and large take-home rations at the upper end of the spectrum. Here we consider some of the key issues in assessing the benefits of school feeding programs versus other forms of social safety nets.

### Adequacy

Safety net programs are most effective if they provide a meaningful level of transfer to the population they are trying to assist. In the conditional cash transfer programs with the largest impacts, the transfer value is of the order of 20 percent of household base income, and social pensions programs often provide transfers of a similar order of magnitude. Less generous programs, including child allowances and programs of last resort, generally provide a transfer that is some 10 percent of household base income (Grosh et al. 2008).

The value of transfer of in-school meals appears to fall in the range of transfer common for other safety net programs. The value of school feeding to the household as a percentage of household base income is rarely reported, but a back-of-the-envelope calculation can give us an approximate range that may be plausible. A family wishes their children to eat three meals a day, or 1,095 meals a year. The school year may be 180 days, and the program will serve one meal per school day. Thus, a child may receive about 16 percent of his or her meals at school. The share in total income for the family will be less, because even poor families must spend on things other than food. Assuming that a generous two-thirds of their expenditure goes to food, and that the schoolchild eats an average amount per person for the family, the program might supply about 10 percent of household expenditure for each child who participates, a not inconsequential sum, especially as some families will have more than one child participating. Furthermore, a study in the Philippines indicates that child caloric intake shows virtually no impact on intrahousehold reallocation of calories, and that in that setting, the individual child benefited from the meal (Jacoby 2002). Take-home rations are not constrained by the amount of food a single child would customarily eat in a single sitting, and so can provide still larger transfers.

### Reaching the Poor

To be effective, safety net programs must reach the poor. School feeding programs face challenges in reaching the poorest wherever enrollment is less than universal because enrollment rates are always lowest among the poorest. The importance of this issue is context specific. In urban Botswana, for example, enrollment is effectively universal and the potential errors of exclusion resulting from children not being in school are hardly a concern. But quite the opposite is true in rural Mali, where fewer than half the children attend school, so in-school feeding programs will potentially miss most of the poorest children and errors of exclusion are large. There are also important gender dimensions, because in many, though not all, settings girls are less likely to be enrolled than boys. These errors of exclusion are likely to increase with age and level of education, because first grade enrollment is always higher than that of higher grades, and by the upper secondary grades, enrollment is often much less than half of first grade enrollment and highly skewed to the better-off children. School feeding programs themselves contribute to enhanced enrollment, so the potential for exclusion may change as the programs are implemented.

Safety net programs also often try to concentrate their benefits on the neediest to provide maximum resources to them within a constrained budget. This leads to the concept that it is an "error of inclusion" to provide benefits to those who are not poor.

Geographic targeting—including some districts or schools but not others—is ubiquitous in school feeding programs. In-school meals are usually served to all children in the school including non-needy children, to avoid issues of logistics, jealousies, or stigma that might arise if only some children are fed. Where such programs are relatively small, geographic targeting can be powerful and result in most of the benefits going to the poor. A program that serves 10 percent of schools and is placed only in the poorest districts would have few errors of inclusion. But as coverage increases and grows toward universal, school feeding programs will include higher portions of nonpoor children. Take-home rations are sometimes targeted to individual households within schools and have the potential to be more finely targeted and have less direct trade-offs between coverage and errors of inclusion. Like most other targeting, however, this may also result in issues of logistics, jealousies, or stigma.

Because of these factors, the distribution of benefits from school feeding programs often favor the poor over the nonpoor; that is, they differentially benefit the poor, but less than programs that use household targeting systems. Figure 3.1 compares in-school feeding, which is geographically targeted, and conditional cash transfer programs in Latin America, which use household targeting systems (often complemented by geographic targeting). The analysis shows that in-school feeding programs are progressive, in contrast to scholarships in this setting, and provide targeting outcomes that are similar to those of other cash and food interventions, but less effective than conditional cash transfer programs. This type of analysis should be used routinely to assess which of the range of possible safety net options is most appropriate in the local context.

There is less comparative evidence elsewhere, and a particular need for studies to explore the performance of social safety net instruments in low-income settings in Africa, where other safety net options, especially conditional cash transfer programs, tend to be small and rare, and where

**Figure 3.1    Targeting Results from Latin America and the Caribbean: School-Related Social Assistance Programs**

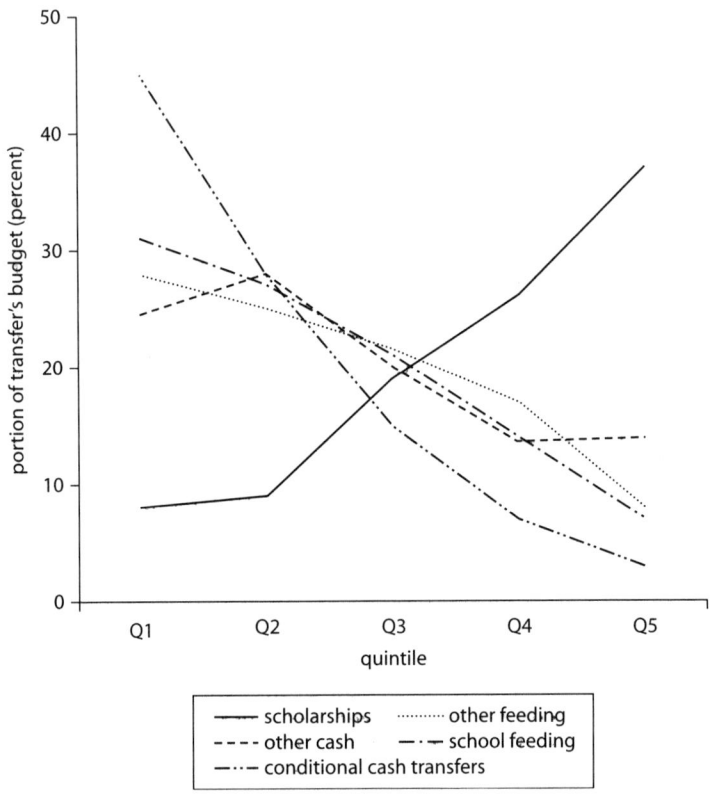

*Source:* Lindert et al. 2006.

*Note:* Absolute incidence of school-related social assistance instruments in Latin America and the Caribbean. Absolute incidence is a measure of the portion of the transfer's budget that reaches each income quintile of the population. Quintile 1 is the poorest, and quintile 5 is the richest.

school feeding programs are often part of a very limited choice of immediately available social protection instruments.

### Cost-Effectiveness
School feeding programs have rather high nontransfer costs compared with other safety net programs. This is largely because all programs must transport and store food, an inherently costly proposition. Programs that serve hot meals must also cook the food, which implies additional labor costs and the provision of at least minimal equipment and infrastructure

for this purpose. These costs can run substantially higher than those for cash transfer programs. Median administrative costs for cash transfers are 9 percent, but 21 percent for all food programs.

The administrative costs of school feeding programs vary by modality. The nonfood costs of on-site meals are quite high as a result of preparation, transportation, and handling. In one analysis, administrative costs were found to account for 30 percent (range 10 percent to 55 percent) of total program costs (Grosh et al. 2008), while an analysis of the costs of programs in Kenya, Lesotho, Malawi, and The Gambia finds administrative costs of 40 percent (Galloway et al. forthcoming). Programs delivering snacks have lower nonfood costs of about 20 percent, according to analysis in Bangladesh, India, and Indonesia (Gelli et al. forthcoming). Take-home rations may have administrative costs of greater than 35 percent (Ahmed et al. 2007) because they require transportation of relatively larger quantities of food and require monitoring of student attendance to determine eligibility, but there is a specific lack of cost data on take-home rations. More details on costs of school feeding programs can be found in chapter 4.

### Incentive Compatibility and Long-Term Benefits

Safety net programs try not to disrupt recipient household's choices about time use and labor in ways that would lower their income. On the contrary, where possible they aim to help households increase their independent welfare. With school feeding programs the objective of increasing independence is sought by encouraging the participation of children in education and, where possible, by promoting their learning. This will not immediately increase household income, and may in fact reduce income by making the children unavailable for work, but in the long run additional schooling should increase the child's income as an adult and help interrupt the intergenerational cycle of poverty. Thus, school feeding programs are among the several safety net programs that can have significant long-term benefits beyond the value of the immediate transfer.

Table 3.1 reviews the key criteria used to judge safety net policy (see Grosh, del Ninno, and Tesliuc 2008 for further discussion of these criteria) and applies them to school feeding programs.

### Take-Home Rations versus In-School Meals

A recurrent theme throughout this consideration of school feeding as social safety net programs is that take-home rations and in-school meals are different in both their inputs and outcomes. Take-home rations can be

**Table 3.1 To What Extent Is School Feeding a Good Safety Net?**

| Criteria | Definition | School feeding modalities (meals, snacks, take-home rations) |
|---|---|---|
| Appropriate | The program responds to the particular needs of a country and is customized to the context. | • All three modalities can respond to the particular needs of a country and be used to customize the program to the context. |
| Adequate | The program should provide full coverage and meaningful benefits to the population it is trying to assist. | • *Meals* benefit schoolchildren directly. The size of transfer can be on the order of 10 percent of base household income or more, and is thus in line with common practice. There may be additional benefits from educational achievement that are not costed. Household benefit would increase with the number of children in school receiving the meal.<br>• *Snacks and biscuits* give benefits similar to those of meals with some differences. The size of the transfer may be less than with meals, and they may have less of an effect on enrollment and attendance.<br>• *Take-home rations* benefit the child and the household that receives the rations. While meals and biscuits are capped in the value of the transfer, the size of the take-home rations may be expanded. |
| Equitable | The program should provide the same benefits to individuals or households that are equal in all important respects (horizontal equity) and may provide more benefits to the poorest (vertical equity). | • *Meals and snacks* are difficult to target on an individual basis, but can be targeted geographically to poor schools.<br>• *Take-home rations* may be targeted individually to reach certain vulnerable groups or households. |
| Cost-effective | The program should run efficiently with the minimum resources required to achieve the desired impact, but with sufficient resources to carry out all program functions well. | • *Meals* programs have high nontransfer costs of around 30 percent resulting from preparation and transport costs.<br>• *Snacks and biscuits* may have lower nontransfer costs than meals, of around 20 percent.<br>• *Take-home rations* appear to have surprisingly high nontransfer costs of around 35 percent. |

| | | |
|---|---|---|
| Incentive compatible | The program should avoid changing households' behavior in a negative way, may even encourage positive changes. | • *Meals* may have significant educational benefits beyond the value of the immediate transfer related to enrollment, attendance, dropout, educational achievement, and cognition.<br>• *Snacks and biscuits* may have similar educational benefits beyond the value of the immediate transfer related to educational achievement and cognition, but lower benefits on enrollment and attendance.<br>• *Take-home rations* may have benefits beyond the value of the transfer on enrollment, attendance, and dropout. |
| Sustainable | The program should be politically and financially sustainable. Programs started with donor support should be gradually incorporated into the public sector. | • *Political sustainability.* Meals have strong political and community support; this is less clear for snacks or take-home rations.<br>• *Financial sustainability.* In low-income countries, the unit costs are highly variable and may provide opportunities for significant cost reduction. Additionally, as per capita income increases in a country, the relative cost of the program decreases. |
| Dynamic | The program should evolve over time as the economy grows. | • *Meals* may be more difficult to change or adapt because of complex management systems.<br>• *Snacks and biscuits* are more amenable to change or improvement.<br>• *Take-home rations* may be more flexible and adaptable, especially for scale-up in crises. |

*Source:* Adapted from Grosh et al. 2008.

more finely targeted, can give higher value transfers, and have lower administrative costs, yet apparently result in increases in enrollment on a similar scale to in-school meal programs. Thus, from a social protection point of view, and depending on context, they may be preferred to in-school meal programs. Take-home rations are considered particularly appropriate in providing support to orphans and vulnerable children, for example. Although take-home rations programs tend to have somewhat higher administrative costs than conditional cash transfer programs, they otherwise offer potential similar to that of these well-evaluated, currently favored tools in social protection (Fiszbein et al. 2009).

Compared with take-home rations, in-school meals tend to be less finely targeted, capped in the value of their transfer, and incur higher administrative costs. From a strictly transfer point of view, meals may therefore be less preferred. But in-school meals have the potential not only to increase enrollment, but to act more directly on learning by reducing hunger and increasing attention during the school day. Therefore, it is critical to understand whether this potential benefit is actually accruing and how large it is, as is explored in the following section.

## The Educational Benefits of School Feeding

School feeding programs can help to get children into school and help to keep them there, through enhancing enrollment and reducing absenteeism; and once the children are in school, the programs can contribute to their learning, through avoiding hunger and enhancing cognitive abilities. These effects may be potentiated by complementary actions, especially deworming and providing micronutrients. The analysis presented here benefited from early work in this area (Levinger 1986, 1996, 2005; Del Rosso and Marek 1996; Del Rosso 1999; Bundy and Strickland 2000) and from three recent reviews (Kristjansson et al. 2007; Adelman, Gilligan, and Lehrer 2008; Jukes, Drake, and Bundy 2008), which arrive at similar conclusions about the direction of the effects. What is less clear is the scale of effect.

Educators seem rarely to participate in these studies, and are notably absent from some of the review teams. Perhaps as a consequence, the education perspective is seldom represented in the literature on school feeding, and education texts seldom address school feeding considerations. We also note that critical interpretation of cognitive and education test outcomes in some reviews might benefit from expertise in psychometrics and education measurement. One particularly important issue with regard to the effect of health on education is that improved health may have educational benefits for the child, for example, enhancing participation and cognition, but whether this then translates into improved educational outcomes will depend upon endogenous factors such as the quality of teaching and the availability of textbooks. Helping children to be more able and available to learn will not improve education achievement unless it is matched by the delivery of quality education. This review was prepared by a multisectoral team to seek to partially redress the traditional sectoral imbalances.

### School Participation

The decision to enroll a child in school and, thereafter, for the child to attend regularly is influenced by many factors, including the perceived value of education, the availability of employment opportunities, the direct and indirect costs of schooling, and the availability and quality of school facilities. Food incentives offered to students, such as school meals, or food incentives offered to families, such as take-home rations (especially for girls, orphans, and vulnerable children), compensate parents for direct educational costs and opportunity costs from the loss of child labor when children go to school.

Implementation of school feeding programs is associated with increased enrollment, particularly for girls. A recent meta-analysis of WFP survey data from 32 countries in Sub-Saharan Africa (Gelli, Meir, and Espejo 2007) grouped 4,000 primary schools according to the type and length of the school feeding program: those with established programs (on-site meals or take-home rations), those with programs of less than 12 months, and those that had yet to initiate a program and so could serve as proxy controls. During the first year of school feeding assistance, absolute enrollment increased by 28 percent for girls and 22 percent for boys. After the first year, enrollment trends varied according to the type of program. When only on-site meals were provided, there was a change only in the first year of the program; after that the rate of absolute enrollment of girls reverted to levels similar to those before implementation. However, in the highest primary grade, with school feeding programs combining on-site feeding and take-home rations, girls' absolute enrollment increased by 46 percent per year, more than twice the yearly increase in the same grade in schools implementing only on-site feeding. The provision of take-home rations appeared to support the progression of girls through the primary school grades, suggesting a reduction in the dropout rate of female students, particularly in the higher primary school grades. An evaluation of India's Mid-Day Meals (MDM) program, the largest school feeding program in the world, found that female school participation was approximately 15 percent higher in schools that provided the MDM program than in schools that did not (Drèze and Kingdon 2001). However, the MDM program did not appear to have a detectable effect on the enrollment of boys.

Evidence from randomized controlled trials also demonstrates increases in attendance and enrollment and a reduction in dropout with in-school feeding. One study in Jamaica gave breakfast to children for a year and found that attendance rose by 2.3 percentage points more than it rose for the control group from a very high baseline, relative to other low-income countries, of around 80 percent (Powell et al. 1998). A randomized controlled trial of a school breakfast program in Peru also found higher attendance rates in treatment versus control schools (Jacoby, Cueto, and Pollitt 1996), and similar results were seen in a study of Kenyan preschool children receiving breakfast, where school participation of students in the treatment group was 8.5 percent higher than in the control group (Vermeersch and Kremer 2004). Combining an in-school snack with micronutrient fortification (iron, iodine, and vitamin A precursor) in primary schools in South Africa (van Stuijvenberg et al. 1999) resulted in a fall in (diarrhea-related) absenteeism from 79 days to 52 days, an increase in attendance of approximately 15 percent. A fortified biscuit program in Bangladesh appeared to have increased net enrollment rates by 10 percent, increased attendance by 1.3 days per month, and reduced the probability of dropping out by 7.5 percent (Ahmed 2004). A systematic review of these and other school feeding studies in low-income countries also found greater attendance for students receiving in-school meals compared with students in control groups (Kristjansson et al. 2007). On average, the per child increase in school attendance was four to six days a year.

Evaluation of take-home rations programs further shows impact on enrollment. In Pakistan (WFP Pakistan 2005), overall enrollment of girls in assisted schools grew 135 percent between 1998/99 and 2003/04, compared with 29 percent in control schools during the same period, and was particularly strong in the first grade of primary school: 211 percent versus 5 percent in control schools. The program also appeared to increase awareness of the benefits of girls' education: before the program started, 48 percent of households did not send any of their daughters to school; afterward, all households educated at least one daughter. Similarly, the take-home rations program in Bangladesh increased girls' enrollment in program schools by 44 percent, and boys' enrollment by 28 percent, while in nonprogram schools, enrollment increased by 2.5 percent during the same period (Ahmed and del Ninno 2002). An analysis of the Bangladesh school feeding program showed the increase in attendance was significant even when taking account of the endogeneity of program participation (Ravallion and Wodon 1998).

In areas with high HIV prevalence, emerging evidence shows that school feeding has the potential of enhancing enrollment, attendance, and progression of orphans and other vulnerable children (Edström et al. 2008). Schools are viewed by UNESCO and UNICEF as centers for care and support for vulnerable children; hence, the enhanced enrollment of orphans and vulnerable children would be seen as a particular advantage of school feeding.

### Cognitive Abilities and Educational Achievement

Having brought more children into school, the challenge is then for children to learn; school feeding programs can also contribute to this. Poor health and poor nutrition among school-age children diminish their cognitive performance either through physiological changes or by reducing their ability to participate in learning experiences, or both. Short-term hunger, common in children who do not eat before going to school, results in difficulty concentrating and performing complex tasks, even if the child is otherwise well nourished.

Students in school feeding programs have the potential for improved educational attainment, as evidenced by results of several randomized controlled trials. A study in Jamaica found scores in arithmetic improved by 0.11 standard deviation(SD) for the youngest children (in grade 2 at the beginning of the study) (Jukes, Drake, and Bundy 2008). Analyses suggested that this improvement was because children attended school more frequently and because they studied more effectively while at school (Simeon 1998). The feeding program did not improve arithmetic in older children or reading and spelling in children of any age. In Kenya, schoolchildren were given milk, meat, or energy supplements for 21 months (Whaley et al. 2003). Children who were given meat improved their arithmetic scores by 0.15 SD and their performance on the Raven's Progressive Matrices Test (a test of nonverbal reasoning) by 0.16 SD, but they did not improve on verbal comprehension. An evaluation of a fortified biscuit program in Bangladesh also found that participation was associated with a 15.7 percent increase in test scores, with particularly strong improvements in mathematics (Ahmed 2004). A study in the Philippines found that school feeding led to improved achievement in English and, when combined with a program to develop parent-teacher partnerships, also improved achievement in mathematics (Tan, Lane, and Lassibille 1999). A study in Uganda found that take-home rations improved mathematics scores for older children and led to an improvement in performance on the Primary Leaving Examination (Adelman, Alderman, Gilligan, and Lehrer 2008). In-school feeding improved mathematics scores for children who had delayed school entry and also led to a slight improvement in literacy scores for all children. Both feeding interventions improved performance on one test of cognitive function. Further evidence comes from a meta-analysis of controlled before-and-after studies, which found a mean improvement in mathematics test scores of 0.66 SD as a result of school feeding programs (Kristjansson et al. 2007).

Because school feeding has the potential to alleviate short-term hunger, the effects of hunger on cognition are also important to consider. In one study in Jamaica, eating breakfast improved scores of malnourished children by 0.25 SD more than the scores of adequately nourished children without breakfast in three cognitive tests of memory and speed of processing and one test of arithmetic taken later that day (Simeon and Grantham-McGregor 1989). The findings suggest that missing breakfast impairs performance to a greater extent for children of poor nutritional status. The results of another trial also indicate that chronically undernourished school-age children are likely to have poorer cognitive abilities. Working with undernourished children in Colombian families of low socioeconomic status, a study found that a program of nutritional supplementation, health care, and education was able to narrow the gap in cognitive abilities between program participants and wealthier peers (McKay et al. 1978).

A study in England addressed the question of whether there are any educational benefits from improvements in food quality for children (Belot and James 2009). As part of Celebrity Chef Jamie Oliver's "Feed Me Better" campaign, primary schools in an area of London shifted from low-budget processed foods toward healthier options. Using a difference-in-difference approach for a comparison with areas that had yet to make the change, the study found significant improvements in English and sciences. This study suggests that food quality affects education outcomes even for children in a rich country who are not undernourished. This may be an important area for future study in low-income settings, especially given the finding from a study in Kenya that meat, but not milk or energy supplements, had an impact on education measures (Whaley et al. 2003).

### Complementary Interventions: Deworming, Micronutrient Fortification of Food, and Micronutrient Supplementation

The analyses above show that school feeding can improve school participation; alleviate short-term hunger; and increase children's ability to concentrate, learn, and perform specific tasks. These effects are not limited to but are greater among children who are also chronically undernourished. If the food is fortified and combined with deworming, there may be additional benefits for children's cognitive abilities and educational achievement.

Evidence suggests that the integration of deworming into school feeding programs has the potential to augment educational benefits. Deworming has significant impacts on school participation; a large randomized controlled trial in Kenya found that treatment increased school participation by 7 percent, amounting to a 25 percent decline in total absence (Miguel and Kremer 2004). A comprehensive review of studies found that schoolchildren infected with worms performed poorly in tests of cognitive function (Watkins and Pollitt 1997). Results from randomized controlled trials show that those heavily infected showed improvements in cognitive function after deworming treatment (Nokes et al. 1992; Grigorenko et al. 2006). The effects of deworming depend on children's nutritional status. A study in Tanzania found that a heavy infection with schistosomiasis delayed reaction time only for those children who were also undernourished (Jukes et al. 2002). Intervention studies have also found that children with poor nutritional status benefit the most from deworming (Simeon, Grantham-McGregor, and Wong 1995). Deworming is exceptionally low in cost—less than US$1.00 per year per child to treat all the common worms—and is among the most cost effective of education interventions (Abdul Latif Jameel Poverty Action Lab 2005; Bleakley 2007).

There is also good evidence linking iron deficiency anemia with poor cognitive abilities in children (Grantham-McGregor and Ani 2001). Further experimental studies with school-age children have found that iron supplementation improves performance on memory, visual/motor coordination, and concentration tests as well as on school exams (Soemantri, Pollitt, and Kim 1985; Seshadri and Gopaldas 1989). Even though many of these improvements are large (approximately 0.5 SD in some cases), the appropriateness of delivering iron supplementation along with deworming should also be considered, given that schistosomes and hookworms contribute to anemia. Vitamin A also affects iron metabolism, and the ease of the pill regimen promotes inclusion of vitamin A supplementation in school-based health programs. The impact of multiple micronutrient fortification, including iron, iodine, and beta-carotene (a precursor of vitamin A), was studied in KwaZulu-Natal, South Africa. Children receiving fortified biscuits for 43 weeks demonstrated improved short-term memory compared with children in the control group (van Stuijvenberg et al. 1999). Because performance on other tests was mixed, multiple micronutrient fortification may be a particularly promising area of research. Both supplementation and for-tification are very low-cost interventions.

As recently highlighted in an assessment of school feeding (Adelman, Gilligan, and Lehrer 2008), despite a large literature on impact, many studies suffer from methodological shortcomings that limit the quality of their contributions, and more carefully designed studies are needed. However, based on the evidence summarized in this section, table 3.2 pro-vides a qualitative assessment of the relative effect of school feeding and complementary interventions. It is clear that all of these actions have effects on key educational indicators. Meals distributed to girls and boys can have relatively higher effects on enrollment of girls than of boys, although this may be context specific (Alderman and King 1998; Dréze and Kingdon 2001). The stronger effects of take-home rations on school access of girls depend on whether they are targeted to girls or other disad-vantaged groups. Both meals and take-home rations increase cognition and educational achievement. While there may be more studies showing this effect with meals, the only two studies (Uganda and Burkina Faso) that compare meals and take-home rations under similar contexts found little

**Table 3.2    An Assessment of the Effect of School Feeding and Complementary Actions on Education Outcomes and Cognitive Abilities**

| School feeding activity | Enrollment | Attendance | Educational achievement | Cognitive abilities |
|---|---|---|---|---|
| In-school meals | + (♀ effect) | +++ | +++ | +++ |
| Take-home rations | + (♀ effect) | + | ++ | ++ |
| Fortified biscuits | + | ++ | + | ++ |
| Supplementation | + | +++ | +++ | +++ |
| Deworming | n.a. | +++ | ++ | ++ |

*Source:* Authors' compilation. See text for data sources.
*Note:* n.a. = Not assessed.
+ = evidence from quasi-experimental evaluation.
++ = evidence from at least one randomized controlled trial.
+++ = evidence from more than one randomized controlled trial.
♀ effect = enhances enrollment of girls.

difference (Alderman, Gilligan, and Lehrer 2008). There is also a paucity of studies examining the relationship between education and fortified foods, which may explain why the relative benefits of fortification versus supplementation are less well understood. Deworming shows its strongest effects on attendance and cognitive abilities, although the impact on enrollment has yet to be directly assessed.

To advise policy makers correctly, there is an urgent need to run long-term randomized controlled trials of school feeding programs in low-income countries and to determine the effects of age and nutritional status of the children, the quality of the education, and the timing of the meal. The special needs of orphans and vulnerable children should also be considered.

## The Nutritional Benefits of School Feeding

The priority in nutrition interventions is to prevent malnutrition during fetal development and the early years of life—the most critical period for growth and development. Thus, the most cost-effective nutrition interventions are those that target the first 24 months of life, and those that promote maternal nutrition and thus intrauterine growth. There is substantial evidence that investing in early nutrition has profound consequences for subsequent development. Early child development programs show significant long-term impacts on subsequent growth and development, including school performance. Similarly, avoidable early deficits have long-term negative consequences.

From this perspective, providing food to school-age children cannot reverse the damage of early nutritional deficits. A schoolchild who is short for age was stunted by inadequate nutrition at an earlier age, and early nutrition intervention would have been required to address this. Although the most recent systematic review shows that providing meals at schools can have a significant impact on the growth of school-age children (Kristjansson et al. 2007), the effect is small and probably cannot reverse the consequences of earlier malnutrition.

There are intergenerational benefits for younger children. The links between school feeding and increased enrollment point to a positive effect on the well-being of the next generation because both maternal and paternal education levels are strong determinants of child growth and development as measured by stunting. The odds of having a stunted child decrease by about 4–5 percent for every additional year of formal education achieved by mothers (Semba et al. 2008).

There is emerging evidence that take-home rations can contribute to enhanced growth of young children, presumably by increasing the availability of food or financial resources in the household. Recent randomized controlled trials of take-home rations programs in Burkina Faso show a significant increase in weight (weight-for-age and weight-for-height z-scores) of children ages 12 to 60 months (Kazianga, de Walque, and Alderman 2009). In these programs, the families were allocated 10 kilograms of meal on condition that the school-age child attended school. Girls of school age and their younger siblings of both sexes exhibited significant improvements in anthropometric measures. There is also evidence from two studies (Ahmed 2004; Lukito et al. 2006) that schoolchildren shared biscuits they received in school with their younger sisters or brothers at home, potentially creating a spillover effect and reaching younger children in some households.

There is good evidence that activities complementary to school feeding, especially deworming and micronutrient supplementation and fortification, can offer important nutritional benefits.

### Micronutrients

Micronutrient deficiency can occur at any age and is common in schoolchildren. For example, estimates suggest that in Sub-Saharan Africa and in India, half of the schoolchildren in poor communities are deficient in iron. Intervention at school age offers direct benefits for the schoolchild, because current micronutrient deficiencies, unlike stunting and other long-term consequences of earlier malnutrition, are rapidly reversible at any age. There are clear nutritional benefits for schoolchildren of providing foods that have been fortified with micronutrients. The recent Uganda studies, for example, found declines in anemia prevalence with both meals and take-home rations (Adelman, Alderman, Gilligan, and Konde-Lule 2008). A randomized placebo-controlled trial in children ages 6–11 years in South Africa showed that fortified biscuits reduced the prevalence of low serum retinol, low serum ferritin, anemia, and low urinary iodine (van Stuijvenberg et al. 1999). Similarly, a randomized placebo-controlled trial in children ages 3–8 years in Kenya showed that iron-fortified whole maize flour improved indicators of iron status (Andang'o et al. 2007). While ensuring the fortification of foods included in school feeding programs presents some logistical challenges (see chapter 4), it is very cost effective.

### Deworming

Infection with common roundworms and bilharzia (schistosomiasis) tends to be most prevalent and intense in children of school age who, therefore, benefit disproportionately from deworming (Bundy 2005). Although it is difficult to detect changes in growth in schoolchildren, because growth has slowed down by this age, there is evidence of growth in randomized controlled trials, as well as evidence for some catch-up growth. Equally important, there is evidence of significant reduction in

**Box 3.1**

## School-Based Deworming: Evolution of an Education Policy Priority

In 2000, the FRESH (Focusing Resources on Effective School Health) framework was launched at the World Education Forum in Dakar, Senegal, with UNESCO, UNICEF, WFP, WHO, and the World Bank among the early partners. The expanded commentary on the Dakar Framework for Action, which describes health as *an input and condition necessary for learning*, and the FRESH framework promoted a core group of cost-effective activities, including deworming, to deliver on the promise of Education for All.

WHO, through a World Health Assembly Resolution in 2001, urged all member states where worm infections were common to attain *a minimum target of regular administration of chemotherapy to at least 75 percent of all school-age children at risk of morbidity by 2010*, recognizing school-based deworming as among the most cost-effective delivery mechanisms.

More recently, Deworm the World (a global coalition of partners launched by the Young Global Leaders of the World Economic Forum) has promoted understanding of the remarkable cost-effectiveness of school-based deworming as an education intervention, and is helping countries to develop large-scale, sustainable, education sector–led programs.

At the 2008 World Economic Forum in Davos, Switzerland, the Executive Director of WFP announced, "The United Nations World Food Programme is scaling up deworming activities to include in all its school-feeding programmes where parasitic worms are a serious problem. In 2008, WFP dewormed 11 million of the 22 million school-age children we feed in school. Deworm the World and WFP will continue to work together to increase coverage to treat an additional 2 million children in 12 more countries in 2009 under WFP assisted school feeding programmes."

In 2009, the Education for All-Fast Track Initiative Secretariat and Partnership are working with all these partners to respond to country demand for quality, school-based deworming programs led by the education sector (http://www.education-fast-track.org).

*Source:* Authors.

anemia with deworming (Gulani et al. 2007; Brooker et al. 2008). The fact that worm infections affect some 500 million schoolchildren argues that deworming can make an additional nutritional contribution if included in the school feeding package. Programmatic evidence suggests that deworming through schools is safe, cheap, and remarkably cost effective (Abdul Latif Jameel Poverty Action Lab 2005; Bleakley 2007), whether implemented as a stand-alone intervention through schools or implemented at the margins of a school feeding program.

## Defining Objectives in Practice: Safety Net, Education, or Nutrition?

In today's world, the primary drivers for increased support for school feeding are the benefits for social protection and for education. The social safety net roles of school feeding programs include an immediate response to social shocks as well as social protection over the longer term. School feeding can benefit education indicators in enrollment, attendance, cognition, and educational achievement, although the scale of benefit and the evidence of effect vary with feeding modality. Well-designed school feeding programs, which include micronutrient fortification and deworming, can provide nutritional benefits and should seek to complement and not compete with nutrition programs for younger children, which remain a clear priority for targeting malnutrition overall.

The focus on school feeding as both a social protection and an education intervention has led to some tensions between the two sectors, but this proves to be a false dichotomy. As we will see in subsequent chapters, the creation of effective safety nets through school feeding programs requires the commitment of a cast of actors that crucially includes the education sector. Policy analysis shows that the effectiveness and sustainability of school feeding programs, whatever their purpose, is dependent upon embedding the programs within education sector policy. The clear education benefits of the programs are a strong justification for the education sector to own and implement the programs, while these same education outcomes contribute to the incentive compatibility of the programs for social protection. Hence, the value of school feeding as a safety net, and the motivation of the education sector to implement the programs, are both enhanced by the extent to which there are also education benefits.

School feeding programs also offer other benefits. For example, appropriately designed programs can make a significant contribution to gender equity in education at the same time as they target the social vulnerability of girls. Similarly, programs can be designed, for example, to provide targeted transfers and strengthen educational access to address vulnerability resulting from disability or the effects of HIV on the household. Apart from these individual, household, and social benefits, there is growing evidence that the programs can help create a stable demand for food at the local level, which, in turn, has important multiplier effects on the local economy and the local community. These issues are explored further in the next chapter.

---

**Box 3.2**

## Case Studies: School Feeding Programs in Transition from Stage 2 to Stage 3
(for further details, see table 4.1)

### Cambodia

The school feeding program in Cambodia reaches about 580,000 children with school meals, and 19,000 children (mostly girls) receive take-home rations (WFP 2007b). The program is implemented as part of the country's Education for All National Plan 2003–2015 and Education Sector Plan 2006–2010 to tackle problems related to high dropout rates, particularly in the upper-primary grades, and low completion rates. In these two sector plans, school feeding is identified as a strategy to improve equitable access to education services for disadvantaged children, especially girls, and improve the quality of education provided.

*Integrating the program into national policy.* A programming mission for the Education for All-Fast Track Initiative to Cambodia in 2007 found that school feeding was the main channel to provide subsidies to poor students in primary schools. Conditional cash transfer schemes focused largely on lower-secondary schools and had limited outreach. However, school feeding depended almost exclusively on WFP for funding and implementation support, and the national Ministry of Education lacked a strategy for school feeding, despite its mention in education sector plans. The mission, therefore, recommended several initiatives to develop a sustainable strategy for cash and food-based incentive schemes in primary education.

### Mali

The government of Mali works predominantly with WFP and Catholic Relief Services (CRS) to support school feeding in the country. During the 2007–08 school year, the school feeding program provided cereal, pulses, and oil that were used to serve hot noontime meals to 108,524 children in 712 rural public elementary schools, which equates to about 8 percent of the nation's school-age children (Lambers 2008).

*(continued)*

**Box 3.2** *(Continued)*

Data indicate that the program has increased attendance and enrollment rates over the years. Of the children enrolled in school, attendance rates for 2007 were above 90 percent for both boys and girls in schools offering school feeding. National school enrollment rates in public and community schools without the program rose 5.9 percent between 2006 and 2007, whereas enrollment in school feeding schools rose 20 percent during the same period, with enrollment for girls increasing 23 percent (Mali Ministry of Basic Education 2008).

*Integrating the program into national policy.* Recently, the Ministry of Education, in collaboration with the Ministries of Agriculture; Health; Water; Social Development; and Promotion of Women, Children and Families; and the Food Security Commission drafted a national policy for school feeding that is currently awaiting a final approval by the Legislative Assembly. The national policy includes a five-year plan to gradually establish 3,000 government-run school canteens. Initially, the government will cover 90 percent of the associated costs, with this percentage decreasing each year as schools and communities become increasingly able to maintain and operate programs (Mali Ministry of Basic Education 2008). The government of Mali has committed approximately US$8 million for school canteens in 2009 using a combination of funds from the national budget and funds from donor countries (Traore and Maiga 2008).[a] The plan includes provisions that support local purchases of commodities, which augments the incomes of smallholder farmers and saves on transport costs.

Information for this case study provided by Rachel Winch, Global Child Nutrition Foundation.

a. Personal interview with Adama Moussa Traore, Associate National Director of Basic Education, and Dr. Bonaventure Maiga, Technical Advisor for the Ministry of National Education.

# CHAPTER 4

# Planning for Sustainability

Any reading of the school feeding literature will show that debate around the sustainability of the programs and the need for an "exit strategy" are recurrent themes (Levinger 1986, 1996, 2005; del Rosso and Marek 1996; del Rosso 1999; Bundy and Strickland 2000; WFP 2003). In this review, we conclude that the concept of a school feeding exit strategy has tended to confound thinking about the longer-term future of school feeding programs. In reality, many countries for which data are available do not seem to seek to exit from providing food to their schoolchildren. On the contrary, many countries appear to seek to expand the coverage of their programs and establish them as national programs mainstreamed into national policy. The aim is not to exit in the sense of closing down the programs, but rather to transition from externally supported projects to national programs. The World Food Programme (WFP) describes 28 countries that have successfully transitioned from reliance on its support (WFP 2007c).

This chapter explores some of the elements of how this has happened, and what this implies for school feeding programs that seek to transition to long-term sustainability. The chapter first explores what we know about the costs of school feeding, and how these relate to economic growth, before examining how school feeding programs have evolved in countries, and what this tells us about the transitional processes. Finally, this chapter describes how the countries that have made this transition have all become less dependent on external sources of food, and examines whether local procurement may offer economic and social benefits.

Three important conclusions emerge. First, programs in low-income countries exhibit large variation in cost, with concomitant opportunities for cost containment. Second, programs become more affordable with economic growth, which argues for focused support to help low-income countries to move through the transition. Finally, the main preconditions for the transition to sustainable national programs are mainstreaming school feeding in national policies and plans (especially education sector plans), national financing, and national implementation capacity. These conclusions suggest that further benefits might accrue from better alignment of development partner support for school feeding with the processes already established to harmonize development cooperation in the education sector, notably the Education for All-Fast Track Initiative (EFA-FTI). A key element of such alignment is ensuring that all new programs are designed within the policy framework of the education sector and that existing programs are revisited so that they do the same. Findings also point to the fact that countries may benefit from having a clear understanding of the duration of donor assistance and a concrete plan of transition to national ownership with time frames and milestones for the process.

## Demand for School Feeding Programs

In considering the elements that make a program sustainable there is a tendency to focus on the issues of cost, logistics, and financing, as indeed much of this chapter does. But a crucially important element of sustainability is the continuity of demand for a program. The importance of demand, even in rich countries, is well illustrated by the recent failure of measles vaccination programs in the United Kingdom, where an exceptionally cost-effective intervention of proven efficacy, with an established universal delivery infrastructure, failed simply because a significant element of the community no longer wanted their children to be vaccinated. This can be contrasted with the public outcry that attended the withdrawal in the 1970s of milk provision in primary schools in England, which became a nationally important political issue despite the lack of evidence for need or impact. Attempts to withdraw or close down school feeding programs in low-income countries, where there is demonstrable impact, have a well-documented history of both social and political reaction. This high level of public demand is an important factor in the sustainability of school feeding programs.

## How the Costs of School Feeding Relate to the Costs of Education

Concerns about cost-effectiveness, costs of food versus education, and the long-term viability of donor-supported programs pervade school feeding policy discussions. Yet we were unable to find data-based analyses of these issues. Here, we obtained data on the per capita costs of school feeding programs (of any modality) and the per capita costs of primary education, and examined how these changed with per capita GDP, as a measure of economic growth (see figure 4.1). The results show, as expected, that the per capita costs increase with GDP. They also show that the per capita costs of school feeding increase much more slowly with economic growth than do the costs of education. It is perhaps worth stressing that the figures as presented tend to minimize this difference, first, because they use a logarithmic scale, and second, because the costs here are for primary education alone—the total per capita education costs in the richer countries would be massively greater if they included the costs of secondary and tertiary education.

Using these data, we can explore the absolute cost per child for school feeding, the ratio between these costs and the costs per child for primary education, and how these variables change with per capita GDP (see figure 4.2). Figure 4.2 shows that there is considerable variation in cost and cost ratio in low-income countries, but that the relative cost of school feeding versus education becomes consistently low as GDP rises.

### The Costs of School Feeding in Low- and Low- to Middle-Income Countries

Figures 4.1 and 4.2 taken together show considerable variation in the per capita cost of school feeding and the ratio between this and the per capita cost of primary education, but largely in the poorest countries. The analysis in figure 4.2 shows that there is an apparent discontinuity around per capita GDP US$2500–2600, with countries below this level showing variation in cost ratios from 5 percent to 120 percent, and data from richer countries being much more consistent at around 10 percent

**Figure 4.1    Changes in the Costs per Child of School Feeding and Primary Education with Economic Growth (per Capita GDP) for 58 Countries**

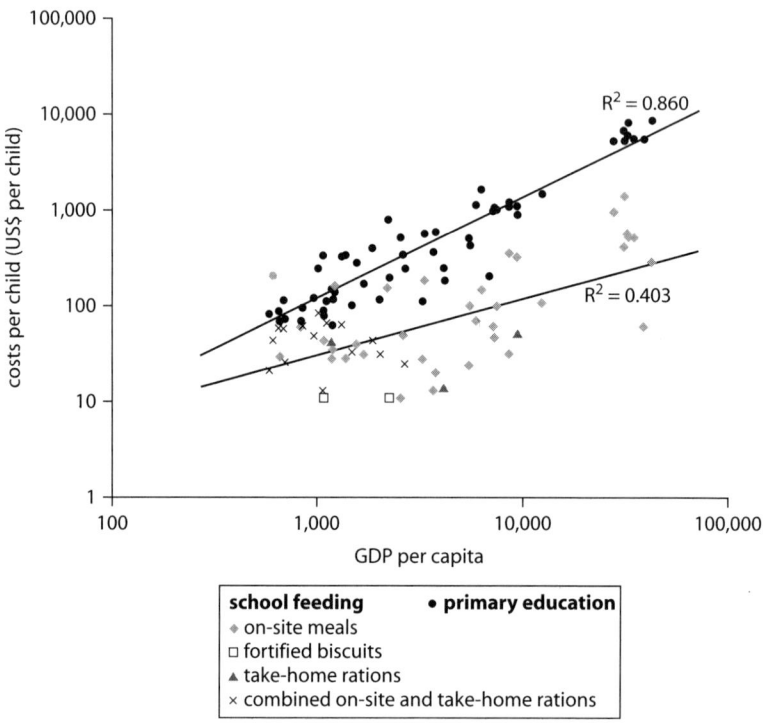

*Source:* Authors. GDP per capita (purchasing power parity, constant 2005 international $) and education costs per child are from the UNESCO Institute for Statistics, and school feeding costs per child were calculated from country program documents and WFP reports. A rigorous search for data was undertaken but it is not claimed that the data are comprehensive.

*Note:* The best fit lines for the school feeding costs and education costs demonstrate how education costs increase more with GDP growth than do school feeding costs. These are logarithmic data so the real differences are greater than they appear. Data are for the same countries. The education data are for primary education only and no attempt is made here to standardize education provision (for example, years of education) between countries. The school feeding costs are per beneficiary estimates, and make no allowance for differences in coverage, which is typically much lower in low-income countries. The costs of school feeding are shown for three different modalities, and one type of combination.

to 20 percent. Note that these analyses are based on per beneficiary costs, and that feeding in low-income countries is typically at levels of coverage of less than 5 percent, whereas basic education will probably benefit more than 50 percent of the population. Thus, the actual per child costs of school feeding, even in these settings, is relatively much lower than for primary education.

This result for the lower-income countries contrasts with the frequent anecdotal claim that per capita school feeding costs are often the

**Figure 4.2    Ratio of per Child Cost of School Feeding in Relation to per Child Cost of Basic Education, versus GDP per Capita**

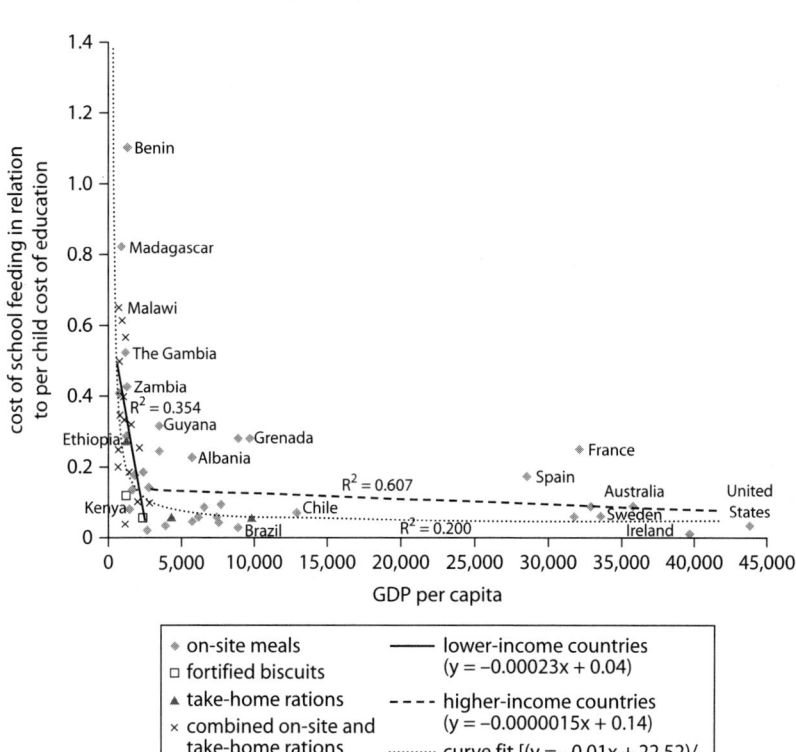

*Source:* Authors. As in figure 4.1, GDP per capita (purchasing power parity, constant 2005 international $) and the education costs per child are from the UNESCO Institute for Statistics, and the school feeding costs per child were calculated from country program documents and WFP reports.

*Note:* In lower-income countries, the cost of school feeding relative to education shows considerable variation, but relative cost tends to be consistent and low in middle-income and rich countries.

The curve fit is the best representation of the relationship between the variables. To fit the curve, linear regressions were made of school feeding cost and education cost per child on GDP per capita. The data are heteroskedastic, so the sums of squares term that was minimized to calculate the best fit was

$$SS = \sum \log(|x - xr|)^2,$$

where $x$ is the value of the school feeding or education cost data point, and $xr$ is the value of the linear regression at this point. The gradient and intercept were varied to minimize this SS. The expression describing the curve fit is the ratio of these regression equations (as shown).

The best fit of the two straight lines highlights the difference between higher- and lower-income countries. To create the two-line fit, the boundary between higher- and lower-income countries was first arbitrarily assigned, and linear regressions were performed either side of the discontinuity, and the least-squares best fit of both lines simultaneously to the data was found. The breakpoint was varied systematically to optimize the fit to data of both lines. The discontinuity between the lower- and higher-income countries was found to be between $2,521 and $2,609 GDP per capita. This corresponds with the 2008 World Bank classification of lower-middle-income countries as those with $936 to $3,705 gross national income per capita.

same as those for education: they certainly are in some countries, and there is one example here where school feeding costs are actually higher than the costs of education, but there are also many examples where the costs of feeding are much lower. This raises the important issue of what causes these differences, apart from the contribution of differing accounting rules. Modality is certainly important, with the costs of biscuits or snacks being much lower than other options, though we only have three estimates here. But this is not the only explanation—the data show that there are meal plus take-home rations programs that are less costly than meals-alone options. The underlying explanation for the cost variation cannot be addressed here, but is clearly a very important area for research given that it implies that there is considerable opportunity for cost containment in precisely those countries where the need is greatest.

### How School Feeding Costs Change with Economic Growth

Per capita costs of feeding relative to education decline nonlinearly with increasing GDP (see figure 4.2). These analyses suggest that the main reason for this is a greatly increased investment per child in primary education as GDP rises, but a fairly flat investment in food. The analyses also show that there appears to be a transitional discontinuity at the interface between the lower- and middle-income countries, which, as we will see from the analysis below, tends to coincide with changes in the capacity of governments to take over the management and funding of programs. Further analysis is required to define these relationships, but an initial conclusion is that supporting countries to maintain an investment in school feeding through this transition may emerge as a key role for development partners. If true, this is a particularly important conclusion because it suggests that external support for school feeding is a transitional and time-bound requirement in national development.

### Cost-Effectiveness of School Feeding: A Critical Need for Impact Studies

Given the potential policy importance of these findings about the cost of school feeding, it is surprising that there appear to be few studies in the published literature that assess and compare the cost-effectiveness and the relative benefits of different modalities of school feeding. There appear to be few evidence-based sources that can help explain why the costs of programs vary so widely among low-income countries, or evidence-based assistance in selecting options to minimize costs.

Recent studies have begun to address this critical gap in the evidence base, and four studies have sought to link costs to outcomes (Ahmed and del Ninno 2002; Ahmed 2004; Ahmed et al. 2007; Galloway et al. forthcoming). However, several factors make comparison difficult: (1) lack of standardization and comparability between programs; (2) the particular lack of small impact studies on take-home rations and fortified biscuit programs; and (3) the lack of standardization of the outcome metrics. This suggests a critical need for cost and impact studies that use a standardized design.

## The Evolution of National School Feeding Programs

In low-income countries there are often major challenges associated with the implementation of school feeding programs. Central concerns are the potential costs of the program and how to implement the program without burdening the already fragile education system. Many countries, especially countries affected by crises, have traditionally addressed these concerns by relying on external support for resources and often the implementation of their programs. A majority of such programs rely on community participation for daily implementation activities, while the overall management of the supply chain is often undertaken by an external partner. Such programs are often peripheral to the education sector management processes and the national budget, and are particularly vulnerable to external factors and may not persist beyond external support. Addressing this vulnerability by building in a plan from the outset that allows for transition to a nationally owned and implemented program is key to long-term sustainability. Evidence from the detailed case study of El Salvador (see appendix 1) suggests that the plan should include an agreement between the government and implementing partners about the duration of external assistance, and clear time frames and milestones for the transition process.

Viewed from this perspective, many of the issues related to school feeding are similar to those faced by education programs more generally: costs, coordination, capacity, and accountability. In education this has led to a move toward a decentralized approach based around school-based management, plans, and budgets. The management of school feeding programs in countries that have successfully transitioned to national support appears to reflect a similar trend.

As countries grow economically, more resources become available and there is typically a concomitant increase in government capacity.

Assessment of the 28 countries with which WFP has direct experience of transition suggests a multistage process from being largely dependent on external resources and implementation, through a transitional stage of mixed government and external financing with external technical and implementation support, to finally becoming a government-run and -budgeted program like any other. In some cases, countries that were largely dependent on external support for their early school feeding programs are now providing technical assistance to other countries for school feeding, as are Brazil, Chile, and India.

Table 4.1 illustrates how programs change as countries evolve through the transition process. For illustrative purposes we give some country examples but recognize that the allocations are necessarily arbitrary, and that some elements of a program may be further along (or behind) the process than others. The situation in specific countries is often complex, particularly where different school feeding models may exist in parallel in a country, and may vary from year to year. Progression from one model to the next may not be linear, especially where social shocks may reverse historical gains. Case study examples throughout this document also illustrate the particularities of programs at different stages of the transition. The discussion that follows seeks to provide guidance on the transition process, but additional case studies of countries that have transitioned would help better define the key elements of a transitional strategy.

## Key Elements of the School Feeding Program Transition Process

Traditional views of the evolution of sustainable programs have focused on increasing the availability of financial resources. The analysis presented here suggests that policy and capacity are also critical elements, and may indeed provide an environment in which resources may more easily be found by governments (see section below on local procurement).

### School Feeding in National Policy Frameworks

An important starting point for any country to begin this transition process is for the government to review the role of school feeding in the development agenda and, where appropriate, integrate the program into the national policy, budgeting, and institutional frameworks, as illustrated in row 1 of table 4.1. In a majority of current programs in stage 1, national policies are largely silent about the role of school feeding. In 70 low-income countries where school feeding programs have been implemented at the request of the government, school feeding is mentioned in 20 of 57

**Table 4.1 The Transition of School Feeding**

| | Stage 1 — Programs rely mostly on external funding and implementation | Stage 2 | Stage 3 | Stage 4 | Stage 5 — Programs rely on government funding and implementation |
|---|---|---|---|---|---|
| Policy framework for school feeding | limited | increased | strong | strong | strong |
| Government financial capacity | limited | moderate | increased | strong | strong |
| Government institutional capacity | limited | limited | moderate | increased | strong |
| Countries | Afghanistan, CAR, DRC, Sudan, Zimbabwe | Malawi, Ethiopia, Haiti, Tanzania, Mali, Cambodia, Rwanda, Niger, Pakistan | Kenya, Côte d'Ivoire, Madagascar, Senegal, Mauritania | Lesotho, El Salvador, Ghana, Ecuador, Honduras | Nigeria, India, Chile, Jamaica, Brazil, Botswana, Namibia |
| Case study examples | Sudan, Haiti (see chapter 6) | Cambodia, Mali (see chapter 3) | Kenya (see chapter 7) | Ecuador, El Salvador (see chapter 4) | India, Brazil (see chapter 2) |

*Source:* Authors, based on information in the WFP database and on discussions with key informants.

*Note:* CAR = Central African Republic; DRC = Democratic Republic of Congo. The allocation of countries to a particular stage is a work in progress.

Poverty Reduction Strategy Papers, and in 23 of 63 national education sector plans. In contrast, all countries in the final stages of transition have well-articulated national policies on the modalities and objectives of school feeding. Indeed, the most developed programs have the highest level of politicization, for example, India where the program is supported by a Supreme Court Ruling, Chile where it is part of a national law and education policy, and Brazil where it is included in the Constitution.

Mainstreaming a development policy for school feeding into national education sector plans is critical to sustainability and offers the added advantage of aligning support for school feeding with the processes already established to harmonize development partner support for education, such as under the EFA-FTI. Integrating the program into national plans may also help attract resources because, with donor harmonization efforts underway, it is increasingly important that school feeding is included in sector plans that form the basis for basket funding or sector-wide approaches that determine the allocation of donor resources. These approaches may help increase the availability of resources allocated, as in row 2 of table 4.1.

Table 4.2 presents an analysis of how school feeding is progressively included in the policy frameworks of countries. Some 32 percent and 25 percent of countries where the school feeding program relies mostly on external funding and implementation (Stage 1) have included the program in their poverty reduction strategies and education sector plans, respectively. As countries increasingly take responsibility for funding and implementing the programs, their policy documents reflect this decision.

**Table 4.2    Countries in Different Transition Stages with School Feeding in Policy Documents**
*(percent)*

|  | Stage 1 | Stage 2 | Stage 3 | Stage 4 | Stage 5 |
|---|---|---|---|---|---|
|  | Programs rely mostly on external funding and implementation | | | | Programs rely on government funding and implementation |
| Poverty Reduction Strategy Paper | 32 | 33 | 38 | 50 | n.a. |
| Education Sector Plan | 25 | 56 | 75 | 100 | 100 |

*Source:* Authors, using data from a WFP database of 57 countries (Svensson 2009) for which information could be confirmed and that could be assigned to a transitional stage. This table is a work in progress.
*Note:* n.a. = Not applicable.

Indeed, it appears that including school feeding in national policy frameworks is one of the preconditions to move from one stage of implementation to the next and toward greater sustainability.

### Government Capacity to Finance School Feeding

Achieving financial sustainability of the program through national resources is another key factor determining the transition. Information from case studies indicates that this is a gradual process involving interim solutions, perhaps with bilateral development partners providing programmatic support. Madagascar and Guyana, for example, recently received funding through the EFA-FTI for school feeding. Ghana secured funding from the Dutch government for its national home-grown school feeding program.

A case study of El Salvador illustrates how countries can also find national sources of funding to carry them through this interim stage (see figure 4.3 and appendix 1). The program was entirely funded by WFP initially, and then was increasingly supported by the interest on a national trust fund established with the proceeds of the privatization of the country's telecommunications company. A law passed in 2000 required that this interest be allocated to social programs, including school feeding. The trust fund has generated about US$32 million for school feeding and in 2008 contributed approximately 30 percent of the total government budget for the school feeding program. During the interim stage the program also received funds from the U.S. Agency for International Development and the U.S. Department of Agriculture. In 2005, the El Salvador Legislative Assembly approved a national budget line for school feeding and institutionalized the program, which in 2008 is entirely supported by the government. Figure 4.3 highlights the last 10 years, but the program started in 1984 and achieved national sustainability in 2008—a transition period of 24 years.

More case studies are needed to shed light on how countries manage to fund a national school feeding program and the different interim solutions that can be found. However, the case of El Salvador illustrates two important points. First, although different sources of external funding can sustain the program until national capacity is in place, there is a need to secure funds from the national budget in the long run. Second, countries appear to benefit from a planned transition process. An initial agreement between the government and donors on school feeding should include a clear understanding of the duration of donor assistance and possible alternatives to external funding as the program evolves.

**Figure 4.3    Yearly Expenditure on School Feeding in El Salvador by Source of Funding, US$**

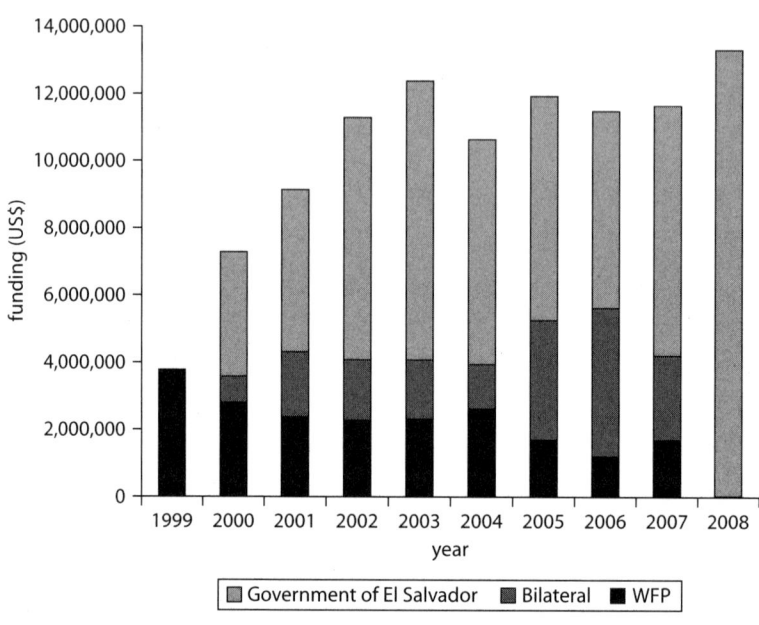

*Source:* Authors, using data from the Ministry of Education of El Salvador.

*Note:* In 1999 the program was entirely funded by WFP. In 2000, other donors began to contribute and the government contributed the proceeds of a trust fund. In 2005 the government established a formal national budget line for school feeding, after which other sources of support were phased out. Today the program is entirely supported by the government budget. See appendix 1 for more details of this case study.

## *Government Capacity to Design and Implement School Feeding*

The implementation of national policies will often require redesign of the program itself, especially where the program has been designed and implemented by external partners and is largely dependent on food aid. There may be a need to reassess ongoing school feeding programs with regard to, for example, relative costs of procuring commodities locally or internationally, long-term implications of substitution for current commodities provided under food aid, and decentralization of implementation arrangements. Redesigning the program may help reduce costs or reduce reliance on foreign exchange.

An additional critical element in these processes is that the government must have the capacity to manage and implement the national program. There are examples of middle-income countries, such as Lesotho, that choose to continue to work with external partners to implement nationally.

Another option is outsourcing to technical partners, as in the private sector program developed in Chile. Whatever the mechanisms, the analysis suggests that full government capacity to actually manage and implement the program in its entirety is often the last part of the process to be completed, as illustrated in row 3 of table 4.1. But for this to happen, the strategies to strengthen the different institutions involved in the program should be planned from the outset and carried out throughout the life of the program.

Case studies show that increasing government capacity for school feeding entails time and a large investment in a variety of capacity development tools (for example, assessments, training, infrastructure, information management systems, and equipment). Capacity development strategies seem to yield better results when they are planned in a systematic way, based on an initial capacity-gaps assessment and on in-depth knowledge of the context and institutional characteristics. Strategies should, therefore, be context specific, properly monitored, and included in the transition agreement between the government and implementing partners. Best practice identifies three levels that are important for capacity development, which should be taken into consideration when designing strategies: the policy and institutional framework, organizations, and individuals (OECD 2006; WFP 2008b).

## Linking School Feeding with Local Agricultural Production

Successful national school feeding programs in middle-income and high-income countries tend to rely on local procurement of commodities, while programs in low-income countries usually find themselves dependent on external sources of food aid. Might this suggest that there is an opportunity here for low-income countries to kick-start their transition, not only establishing sustainable sources for some of their commodities but also contributing to local economic development? African governments clearly think so, and in 2003 included locally sourced school feeding programs in the Comprehensive Africa Development Programme. That same year, the New Partnership for Africa's Development, together with WFP and the Millennium Project Task Force on Hunger, launched a pilot Home-Grown School Feeding and Health Programme designed to link school feeding to agricultural development through the purchase and use of locally and domestically produced food. Because school feeding programs run for a fixed number of days a year (on average 180) and normally have a predetermined food basket, they provide the opportunity to benefit local farmers and producers by generating a stable demand for their products.

A dozen pilot countries (Angola, Democratic Republic of Congo, Ethiopia, Ghana, Kenya, Malawi, Mali, Mozambique, Nigeria, Senegal, Uganda, and Zambia) were invited to implement the program; Ghana and Nigeria have rolled out programs. These programs are being evaluated. For example, the program in Osun State, Nigeria, provides three eggs per week to each schoolchild and a forthcoming study, supported by the Bill & Melinda Gates Foundation, will examine the impact on the local poultry industry. In 2009, the U.S. Department of Agriculture will undertake studies in five African countries to determine the feasibility of purchasing locally for national school feeding programs. WFP is currently testing this approach in its own operations under its Purchase for Progress initiative, which may shed some light on the main knowledge gaps (WFP 2008a).

While awaiting the outcome of these studies, here we examine the current evidence for the economic impact of this approach.

### Evidence from Middle- and High-Income Countries for a Return on Local Procurement

Many high- and middle-income countries are already applying this approach. In the United Kingdom, the East Ayrshire local authority initiated a pilot school meals program in 2004 in 12 schools. Two of the stated objectives of the program were to (1) localize the food chain and repatriate expenditure on food directly into the local economy, and (2) increase the potential for public money to assist sustainable businesses and local employment by procuring the food for the program locally. At present, 70 percent of the food is locally sourced and the 12 schools in the scheme benefit the local economy by US$320,000 per year at the average exchange rate for 2007 (Sonnino 2007).

A background paper for the Millennium Project Task Force on Hunger describes how a locally sourced school feeding program in Guatemala shifted its acquisition of food from centralized industrial suppliers to local producers and helped develop local markets (Caldes and Ahmed 2004). An economic stimulus program initiated during the 1990s economic crisis in Indonesia, and which included only locally produced food, showed evidence of increased sales by local farmers (Studdert et al. 2004). In Chile, where the government initiated a local purchase scheme for school feeding following a natural disaster in the southern part of the country in 2001, local farmers that received support from the National Agricultural Promotion Agency now supply nearly all of the national school feeding program's vegetable requirements in that region (for more details see http://www.junaeb.cl/). In certain contexts, the added demand can also help promote national and local processing capacity, as has been the case, for example, in Malawi, the Lao People's Democratic Republic, and Ghana, where local industries produce a fortified corn-soya blend for the program.

There are reservations about including liquid milk in school feeding programs in low-income countries because of the limited evidence that milk improves the impact of meals. Given its cost and frequent ties to political influence, inclusion of liquid milk should be treated with caution. Furthermore, the high costs of transportation and packaging, and the package waste created, present additional problems (WFP 2007a). But in Asia there are good examples of the contribution of school feeding programs to the expansion of dairy programs. In China, the National School Milk Program created 223 new jobs for every 100,000 children during its initial pilot stage, and in Thailand national milk production increased from 120,000 liters a day to 1,550,000 after the establishment of a national school milk scheme, creating an estimated 250,000 jobs in the dairy industry (Caldes and Ahmed 2004). The benefits for the school-children are not reported.

### Modeling Local Procurement in Sub-Saharan Africa

There appear to be no empirical data on the local returns to school feeding programs in Sub-Saharan Africa, but there have been two economic modeling exercises. The first, commissioned by the Millennium Project Task Force on Hunger, concluded that if demand from school feeding programs induced farmers in Sub-Saharan Africa to switch to modern maize production, the total incremental benefit of supplying the programs with locally produced food was potentially US$1.6 billion a year at 2003 prices, of which 57 percent would go to consumers and 43 percent to producers (Ahmed and Sharma 2004). A more recent modeling exercise done by WFP, in partnership with the International Food Policy Research Institute and the Gates Foundation, estimated the potential benefits of a local purchase scheme in Kenya (Brinkman et al. 2007). The study concluded that if the school feeding program in Kenya were to purchase maize from smallholder farmers in a high-potential area for maize, the annual incomes of 175,000 farmers would increase by around US$50 per smallholder.

An important consideration is whether local purchase schemes are more or less expensive than buying internationally. The Kenya study concludes that lower commodity costs to the program—because local maize prices are lower than international prices—would partially offset higher administrative costs of procuring locally, but that if farmers cannot increase their yields, local purchase schemes might cause a rise in prices, which would harm many net buyers in the region. A recent Food and Agriculture Organization discussion paper reviews the potential for social protection programs to support small farmer development and concludes that food-based social transfers, including school feeding, have the potential to promote rather than inhibit agricultural growth, provided that food is sourced locally and impacts on markets and production are closely monitored (Devereux et al. 2008).

### Overambitious Expectations for School Gardens?

In some countries there are expectations that school feeding programs can be sustained with food grown in school gardens and cultivated by children during school hours. This is understood in some cases as a way to use local agricultural production for school feeding and as a strategy to increase the sustainability of the program. While the participation of children and of communities is certainly a determinant factor in the sustainability of any program, the school garden approach raises some major concerns. First, expecting children and their teachers to grow food on a production scale is exploitative and an inappropriate use of the education system. Second, the practice has potentially serious negative implications for education and cannot be reconciled with the educational aspirations of school feeding programs. Third, the level of production of any normal school garden will be insufficient to sustain an appropriate program. For all these reasons, much more convincing evidence is required before school gardens could be considered part of school feeding operations, except perhaps for educational purposes (see chapter 6).

### Implications for Planning School Feeding Operations Today

The available evidence indicates that local purchase schemes have the potential to yield significant benefits, and already have been shown to do so in high- and middle-income countries. The ongoing studies of the potential benefits of local procurement in Africa will provide much-needed empirical evidence of the benefits of this approach for low-income countries, and guidance on implementation.

For the policy maker it is already clear that this is a model worth exploring, and it might be anticipated that more countries will seek to examine the role of local procurement in their local context. In chapter 5 we offer some guidance on the implementation challenges and the role of the private sector based on the limited experience to date. The private sector may play an important role in enhancing the sustainability of school feeding programs and making the link with national production. Public-private partnerships, both for the local production of food and for the management of the program, emerge as an opportunity that should be explored.

One key point revealed by the theoretical analyses is that the potential gains are only possible if small farmers achieve a higher yield for their crops, which, in turn, requires support through agricultural reforms. The design of local purchase schemes for school feeding, therefore, needs to be linked with local efforts to boost agricultural production.

---

**Box 4.1**

## Case Studies: School Feeding Programs in Transition from Stage 4 to Stage 5
(for further details, see table 4.1)

### *Ecuador*

The school feeding program in Ecuador has evolved over a period of 20 years from initially relying on WFP financial and management support to being a nationally funded program. In 1987 WFP began providing school feeding services for children living in poor and underdeveloped areas; two years later, the government established an operational unit to institutionalize the project under the Ministry of Education. In 1999, school feeding was reaching 667,000 school-age children in 3,000 schools in poor rural areas; the government provided 80 percent of the food. By 2004, Ecuador school feeding programs were exclusively financed by the government.

*Increasing government capacity to manage the program.* The government currently receives external technical support at the policy and implementation levels to improve operational management of the program. Through a trust fund, the government relies on WFP as a service provider for procurement and logistics. Institutionalizing school feeding and promoting participation of mothers were two factors that enabled large-scale implementation of the program that now reaches 2 million children—15 percent of the population—in all 22 provinces in Ecuador (WFP APR 2006a).

*(continued)*

**Box 4.1** *(Continued)*

## *El Salvador*

In 2008, the school feeding program in El Salvador was fully taken over by the government after 24 years of partnership with WFP. The program started during the country's internal crisis in 1984, reaching 300,000 students, 90 percent of school-age children in rural areas. In 1997, six years after the signing of the peace accords, the government began to take over program management responsibilities while WFP withdrew from departments not classified as most food insecure.

*Increasing government capacity to finance and manage the program.* In the early days, most of the financing for government programs came from a trust fund generated through a national privatization initiative. Later, the national school feeding program was financed through increasingly regular government budget allocations. The program was included within the broader National School Health Program, which, in turn, is at the center of the country's social safety net system. By 2006, government allocations totaled US$10 million, reaching 651,260 children in 3,500 schools. Coverage at the national level reached 88 percent of rural primary schools and poor urban schools. The government achieved 100 percent coverage in 2008, coinciding with the planned date for the complete transfer of responsibilities to national institutions (WFP APR 2006b). Currently, the government receives external support for technical assistance, logistics, and procurement through a trust fund that was established in 2008. Through this agreement, WFP is piloting procurement innovations under its corporate Purchase for Progress initiative, which aims to link local procurement with the school feeding program.

*Note:* See also Appendix 1.

# CHAPTER 5

# Trade-Offs in Program Design: Targeting, Feeding Modalities, and Costs

The sustainability and effectiveness of school feeding programs can be optimized by evidence-based decisions about the design of the program. The previous chapter emphasized the importance of designing long-term sustainability into programs from their inception, and of revisiting programs as they evolve. In this chapter we examine how program objectives can be met through careful selection based on the objectives of the program and trade-offs between different targeting approaches, feeding modalities, and costs. As far as possible, given the limited current evidence base, we seek to provide empirical evidence of the costs associated with these choices.

## Approaches to Targeting Programs

Given a finite budget, targeting is essential to ensure that programs provide the most benefits to the intended beneficiaries (see also chapter 3). Before defining the target, an important first step for the government is to define the objective. Where the objective is to tackle gender disparities in access to education, the target is likely to be girls, especially in the higher grades. Where it aims to sustain or strengthen education for the most vulnerable, the target could be, for example, orphans and vulnerable children or in some cases boys. In each case, the objective of the program defines the target population.

In high- and middle-income countries free school meals are generally integrated within social protection programs targeted to individual children on the basis of vulnerability and means-based proxies. Children not considered at risk would normally pay for the meal, though often at subsidized cost. In contrast, the majority of school feeding programs in low-income countries tend to be limited in geographical scope and to target children living in vulnerable, food insecure contexts. Certain school feeding programs combine both forms of targeting offering on-site feeding to all pupils in schools in food insecure areas and also providing take-home rations to vulnerable children (for example, girls in areas with large gender inequality or vulnerable children in the context of HIV). Here we consider some of the targeting approaches used in practice.

### Geographical Targeting

Geography is the most frequent explicit criterion for targeting school feeding programs. Programs may be offered in some schools or districts and not in others. A poverty and food insecurity map, whether crude or sophisticated, informs decisions about the locations where school feeding programs operate. Sometimes, in addition to the geographic location, school characteristics that correlate with poverty are used. For example, preference might be given to schools with multigrade classrooms where these tend to serve the poorest; conversely, private schools might be excluded where they tend to serve the richest. Where school feeding programs are relatively small, geographic targeting can be powerful and can result in most of the benefits going to the poor. A program that serves 10 percent of schools and is placed only in the poorest districts would have few errors of inclusion. But as coverage increases and grows toward universal, school feeding programs will include higher proportions of nonpoor children.

In low-income countries, school feeding programs are targeted on the basis of food insecurity as well as on an analysis of the educational context in each country to identify the areas with greatest educational need. A tool developed by the World Food Programme (WFP) is Vulnerability Analysis and Mapping (VAM), which analyzes the causes of food insecurity and vulnerability among populations affected by conflict, natural disasters, financial or other shocks, or chronic vulnerability (see appendix 2). The analysis usually involves both primary and secondary data collection.

Subnational units such as regions, provinces, or districts are profiled on vulnerability, educational need, and food insecurity. HIV prevalence and rates of orphanhood are added to the criteria to ensure a proper response to HIV through the program. As the targeting becomes more detailed during the design of the program, vulnerability data are usually complemented by information related to future implementation such as security, accessibility and state of schools, coverage of complementary services, availability of partners, and opportunities to purchase food locally.

Urban areas are sometimes overlooked when poverty and food insecurity are assessed geographically because the lowest level of geographical targeting is often the district level. This can result in rural areas being identified as generally worse off, even though increased urbanization and the rapid growth of slum areas in cities have led to urban areas with large populations living in extreme poverty. In such conditions, school feeding programs can be introduced to support vulnerable children.

Once target areas have been identified, the next stage in the process involves school-level targeting. In this process, selecting some schools and not others in a particular area might attract students from neighboring schools, which are not receiving food, to those that are targeted under the program. To avoid this, all or most schools in an administrative or catchment area are usually targeted. Schools in target areas are generally screened on the basis of implementation criteria, sometimes referred to as "minimum standards" (for example, parental interest and support for school feeding and school infrastructure). The minimum standards are developed in collaboration with all stakeholders and depend on context and details of the intended school feeding program. However, schools that do not meet the minimum standards may often be those serving the most vulnerable communities; this tension is often resolved by integrating the necessary support for infrastructure and capacity building as part of the school feeding program implementation.

### Individual Targeting

Different forms of proxy means testing have been developed to target school feeding assistance to individual children on the basis of vulnerability and well-being indicators. Targeting criteria are context dependent, and involve inputs from multiple stakeholders at different levels. Decentralized targeting at the village level was found to be effective in Bangladesh (Galasso and Ravallion 2005). The systems and data requirements for individual targeting are fairly resource intensive and to date have generally been considered out of scope for most low-income countries, though there are effective examples of national programs in middle- and high-income countries.

The national program in Chile is considered an example of good practice regarding individual targeting, not least because the targeting mechanisms have been evolving since the 1960s, reflecting a deeper understanding of the drivers of poverty and educational exclusion. Schools are provided free school meal allocations on the basis of a school vulnerability index built on socioeconomic household data of first grade schoolchildren. Teachers are then asked to target free meal allocations to the most vulnerable children in the classroom; other children in the class get meals but at a cost. This is an interesting alternative to geographic targeting, allowing fewer inclusion errors when scaling up programs.

While targeting individual children on the basis of need can have considerable benefits in cost-effectiveness, it has potential social costs from stigmatization. In certain contexts, beneficiaries of targeted school feeding assistance have been marginalized by other children not being assisted. Strong buy-in from the community is needed to ensure that the negative effects of individual targeting are minimized.

There may be a small element of self-selection pertaining to food served at school, though the results are not well quantified. If food is plentiful at home, and the school lunch or snack is monotonous and bland, some children may choose not to eat the food provided. Field reports of complaints of monotony are common, though if school days are long, children may eat even if they complain. It would also seem that where second servings are allowed, these might favor the children who have eaten less at home, faced the longest walk to school, or have done the most labor before attending and thus be well targeted. Offsetting this, the older children and the bigger ones for any age will have more capacity to eat and are more likely to be better off. Unfortunately, no empirical evidence is known that sheds light on the targeting implications of the distribution of second servings.

## Operational Implications of School Feeding Modalities

As described in chapter 3, there are real differences between the benefits of in-school feeding (meals or biscuits) and take-home rations. The choice of school feeding modality, therefore, depends on program objectives. Similarly, there are significant differences in the appropriateness of the different modalities to local capacity and contexts. Some of the important trade-offs are explored below.

### In-School Meals

The timing and composition of school meals depends on such local factors as the length of the school day, the nutritional status of children, local eating habits, availability of commodities (for example, in the case of in-kind donations), ease of preparation, shelf life of different commodities, and costs, as well as on the availability of trained cooks, cooking facilities, and clean water. Cooking food in school involves the complications and costs of providing labor, fuel, and cooking and eating facilities. These complications are offset somewhat by the fact that they draw parental and community involvement into the program and may include food that is available locally, key elements of quality and sustainability.

The composition and nutritional content of the meal are generally designed in consultation with nutritionists with knowledge of local conditions, habits, and preferences, and depend on the duration of school days. In general, the energy content should reflect the following: (1) half-day school, 30–45 percent of daily requirement (555–830 kcal); (2) full-day school, 60–75 percent of daily requirement (1,110–1,387 kcal); and (3) boarding school, 85–90 percent of daily requirement (1,570–1,665 kcal).

A typical school meal provided for a half-day school for example, may offer 150 grams (g) of cereal, 30g of pulses, 5g of oil, and 4g of salt (about 695 kcal). However, without the inclusion of appropriately fortified commodities, these meals are poor sources of important micronutrients, thus fortification has an important complementary role. If short-term hunger is a problem, the meal needs to be provided in the morning, or when children arrive at school, to increase children's ability to concentrate and learn.

With regard to liquid milk (compared to dry skimmed) as an element in the food ration, there are particular challenges to be addressed (WFP 2007a). These include the high cost of packaging and transporting liquid milk, hygiene considerations, and the waste associated with disposing of the used packaging.

To the extent possible, food should be fortified with minerals and vitamins to benefit nutritional and learning outcomes. Imported foods are normally fortified at source, but foods purchased locally can also be fortified if processing units are available. Examples of countries that produce fortified products for use in school feeding programs are Ghana, Guatemala, Kenya, Lao PDR, Malawi, and Zambia, which all produce corn-soya blend. Fortified biscuits are produced in Bangladesh, the Arab Republic of Egypt,

India, Indonesia, Malawi, and Pakistan, and micronutrient powders are produced in Afghanistan, Cambodia, and Tanzania.

When local capacity to process and fortify foods is lacking, fortification at the point of use and just before consumption is an emerging technology. Micronutrient powder has been used mainly in food-based programs in emergency situations (that is, supplementary feeding) and has been piloted for school feeding in Cambodia and Tanzania (Hamdani 2008). In both countries, the program relied on children sprinkling the micronutrient powder on their own plates of food, which caused delays in eating times and created problems with package disposal. To simplify the process, the product is now being piloted with multidose packaging that can be sprinkled on food by cooks before serving, reducing the cost from US$0.025 per sachet per child to US$0.0045 per dose per child.

### Fortified High-Energy Biscuits and Snacks

Fortified high-energy biscuits may have similar educational benefits to in-school meals but do not require the local costs for food preparation and serving (see box 5.1). Biscuits are typically manufactured centrally and distributed to schools, and are usually packed in individual packets that can be easily stored and distributed. They can also be made locally, as has been shown in The Gambia (Ceesay et al. 1997). Their distribution is usually less disruptive to the school day than cooked meals. To support learning in the classroom, biscuits tend to be delivered as snacks early in the school day. Where children are in school for a full day, the biscuits or snacks may be served in addition to a meal.

School feeding programs that use fortified biscuits have a potential advantage over conventional on-site feeding because a biscuit may be regarded as a snack rather than a meal, and may be less likely to replace meals given to the child at home. While this is a commonly repeated anecdote, we were unable to find evidence for this contention.

Biscuits are not always the preferred choice for children, not least because they are usually not what children normally eat at home. In some cultures, biscuits may not be regarded as proper food and children might thus consider that they have not eaten. When biscuits are very dry children need to be able to drink water to enhance palatability, which may be a concern in schools without safe water. Efforts to enhance palatability by sweetening biscuits may lead to unhealthy eating practices. Moreover, if school access is to be improved along with learning, biscuits may not have sufficient economic and, thus, incentive value, although a well-designed study using biscuits in Bangladesh showed incentive and learning potential comparable to meal programs and at lower cost (Ahmed 2004).

**Box 5.1**

## Case Studies: Evaluated Programs Using Fortified Biscuits

### Indonesia

From 2006 through April 2008, a school feeding program in Indonesia assisted more than 530,000 children in nearly 3,000 primary schools in the most vulnerable areas of Aceh, Greater Jakarta, East Java, Nusa Tenggara Barat, and Nusa Tenggara Timur. The program combined the distribution of fortified biscuits with health, hygiene, and nutrition education through improved teaching materials, and used participatory and fun learning methods. The biscuits were locally produced and fortified and approved by the Indonesian Ministry of Health. They were distributed by cooperating partners on a monthly basis from warehouses to the participating schools. Teachers were responsible for the distribution of the biscuits in the classrooms, and for the provision of nutrition education.

The Southeast Asian Ministers of Education Organization Tropical Medicine Network, the Regional Center for Community Nutrition of the University of Indonesia, Airlangga University, and WFP evaluated the school feeding program. Results of the 2007 survey showed no significant improvement in anthropometric indicators. However, a significant improvement from baseline tests was found in hemoglobin concentration, resulting in decreased anemia prevalence. Median cognitive performance expressed as the percentage of maximum test scores increased significantly for verbal fluency, visual processing, and concentration. In coordination with the local health authorities, there were two rounds of deworming activities in Nusa Tenggara Barat and Nusa Tenggara Timur provinces with coverage at 89 percent.

The cost of the program in 2006 was US$17.59 per child per year.

The program was implemented in coordination with the School Health Coordination Board under the Ministry of Education, with support from WFP.

### Bangladesh

A school feeding program in Bangladesh provides a daily snack of fortified high-energy biscuits to 400,000 students in government and nongovernmental organization (NGO) primary schools in targeted vulnerable and food-insecure areas. Food aid earmarked for school feeding is bartered (monetized) against locally produced fortified biscuits, which are then delivered to and stored by NGO service providers at district warehouses. The NGOs are also responsible for preparing delivery plans; checking attendance and distribution; and inspecting the schools for good storage practices, hygiene, and sanitation. The program is implemented through the Directorate of Primary Education under the Ministry

*(continued)*

**Box 5.1** *(Continued)*

of Primary and Mass Education. For each school, a school management committee (SMC), consisting of parents, teachers, and school officials, oversees the distribution process.

The International Food Policy Research Institute (IFPRI) evaluated the impact of the program (Ahmed 2004). The school feeding program raised gross school enrollment rates by 14.2 percent (10 percent increase in net enrollment rates), reduced the probability of dropping out of school by 7.5 percent, and increased school attendance by about 1.3 days a month. The calories consumed from the biscuits were almost entirely (97 percent) additional to the child's normal diet. Average energy intake of participating students was 11 percent and 19 percent higher in rural and urban slum areas, respectively, than energy intake of primary school students in corresponding control groups. Participating students also appeared to share the biscuits with younger siblings, and energy from the biscuits accounted for 7 percent of total energy intake of children ages 2 to 5 years in beneficiary households in the rural area. The body mass index (BMI) of participating children increased by an average of 0.62 points, a 4.3 percent increase compared with the average BMI of schoolchildren in the control group. Participation in the school feeding program increased test scores by 15.7 percentage points, with particular improvement in math tests. The cost of providing biscuits was under US$12 per child per year.

The program is implemented by the Ministry of Education with support from WFP.

*Source:* Authors.

Through fortification, biscuit snacks can be an important source of micronutrients. In sufficient quantity, biscuit snacks can be a valuable source of nutrients. Biscuits can be fortified with vitamin A, iron, folate, iodine, and sometimes B-vitamins at a level of about two-thirds of daily requirements per serving. The typical nutritional composition of biscuits is some 450 kcals and 12g of protein per 100g of biscuits. However, insufficient quantities of these biscuits provide only a small fraction of the daily recommendations for energy, protein, and fat.

The "blended" food snacks, such as corn-soya blend, are relatively high in protein and can provide enough energy (carbohydrates and fat) if sufficient amounts of blended food, sugar, and oil are provided. The overall micronutrient profile of blended food snacks is the most important attribute because they are well fortified with iron, zinc, and other micronutrients.

Given the limited energy content of biscuits, full-day schools could consider providing a meal in addition to a mid-morning snack to make a significant contribution to the diet.

Provision of snacks presents opportunities for creating local jobs and profits, especially for small or medium bakeries and food processors—even if the ingredients must be imported.

### Take-Home Rations

Take-home rations have the main benefit of being readily targeted to individual groups suffering particular educational disadvantages, such as girls, herdboys, or orphans and vulnerable children, and function rather like conditional cash transfer programs. The size of the rations can be expanded to increase the value of the transfer to households. They are less complex to implement than conventional school meal programs that require substantial investments in both infrastructure and community inputs, but may have certain drawbacks for the same reasons; little community and parental involvement in the school itself, fewer opportunities for job or profit creation, less direct impact on short-term hunger and learning of the students. Food rations are individual and conditional upon regular school attendance, typically at least 80 percent monthly attendance rate.

Take-home rations are a resource transfer and their content is determined by local conditions regarding the value of commodities and availability and ease of storage and distribution. Take-home rations typically use high-value, low-volume commodities such as 10kg sacks of maize or other cereals or 4-liter cans of vegetable oil. Distribution typically takes place once per month or per school term (every three months).

### Combining Different Modalities

In some contexts, school feeding programs combine on-site meals or snack programs with an extra incentive from take-home rations targeting a specific group of vulnerable children identified in the problem analysis; for example, orphans and vulnerable children in the context of HIV, herdboys and other marginalized groups, or girls in higher grades at particular risk of dropping out. By spreading the extra costs of the take-home rations across all the assisted population, benefits to targeted vulnerable groups can be achieved at relatively small additional cost. Based on WFP data, on average, a program that includes on-site meals and take-home rations would typically provide both modalities to about 20 percent of children, with the remaining 80 percent receiving only on-site meals. However, the actual proportion of children receiving both modalities varies considerably from country to country, reflecting the targeted, context-specific nature of the extra take-home rations assistance.

## Costs of School Feeding Modalities and Food Choices

Generally, the costs of school feeding programs will depend on several different factors, including the choice of modality, the composition and size of the rations, whether the food is purchased locally or is imported, and the number of beneficiaries and school feeding days per year. Logistics, security, and climatic conditions have an impact on program expenditures. The geographical context will also affect the overall cost; programs in landlocked countries will generally face greater operational costs than countries implementing the same type of program but that have access to seaports, depending on the provenance of the food.

### In-School Meals

Estimating the full cost of on-site meal programs is not always straightforward because providing cooked meals in schools generally includes a range of school-level costs that are normally not included within overall program expenditures. A recent study estimated the full costs of on-site meal programs by collecting data from school feeding program implementers at all levels in four countries in Sub-Saharan Africa: The Gambia, Kenya, Lesotho, and Malawi (Galloway et al. forthcoming). Program costs were standardized using a typical 200-feeding-day school year and a 700-kcal daily ration, and adjusted for breaks in the food delivery pipeline. The costs of school feeding ranged from US$28 to US$63 per child per year (weighted average US$40 per child per year). On average, commodity costs accounted for 59 percent of the total expenditure. The contribution from local communities averaged 5 percent of the total cost (varying from 0 percent in Lesotho to 15 percent in Kenya), or about US$2 per child per year on average. WFP-estimated costs, which may include some commodity costs, accounted for some 60 percent of the total program costs.

Another study, which estimated WFP project expenditures (that is, the costs of the program to WFP), found that in 19 countries providing on-site meals, the average cost of the program, standardized using the parameters outlined above, was US$20.40 per child per year (Gelli, Al-Shaiba, and

Espejo forthcoming). Regional variations in the costs were mostly due to the choice of school feeding basket choices. Assuming that WFP-estimated costs account for a 60 percent share of total implementation costs, as in the Galloway et al. study, would imply that the full costs for on-site meals would be approximately US$34 per child per year.

### Fortified Biscuits

Because the main inputs for biscuits once they reach the school are storage and distribution to the children, school-level costs for biscuit programs may be considered negligible. A recent full cost analysis of WFP-assisted programs in three countries (Bangladesh, India, and Indonesia) found that the weighted-average standardized cost of providing fortified biscuits was US$12.77 per child per year (Gelli et al. 2006). The cost per beneficiary varied substantially from one country to another, ranging from US$10.86 in Bangladesh to US$17.59 in Indonesia. The cost of commodities accounted for an average of 81 percent of total project costs, 22 percentage points higher than for in-school meals. The Bangladesh study cites a figure of US$18.00 per child per year, for a 240-day year without the above standardization (Ahmed 2004). More work is required to understand the full cost implications for school biscuits throughout the developing world, especially in Sub-Saharan Africa.

### Take-Home Rations

Costs at the school level for take-home rations programs are related to monitoring attendance; no on-site preparation is required. An analysis of the full cost of the take-home rations program in Pakistan found that the full cost of implementing the program, adjusted over breaks in the food pipeline, was US$63 per child per year (Ahmed et al. 2007). Food costs accounted for 63 percent of the total program expenditure.

An analysis of WFP program costs in four countries (China, Ghana, Pakistan, and the Republic of Yemen) found that the average cost of take-home rations was US$52 (Gelli, Al-Shaiba, and Espejo forthcoming). The higher costs for take-home rations compared with other modalities of school feeding were found to be mostly due to the larger volumes of food distributed per child; in this data set, over a school year, take-home rations delivered approximately twice as much food per child compared with on-site meals because the rations are incentives for the household, and the amount and composition most often are determined by the value of the commodity as an incentive, and by average family size. Moreover, the standardization methodology used in this analysis might not always be appropriate for the take-home rations program, where food is distributed conditional on school attendance.

### Cost-Efficiency Considerations in Selecting Feeding Modalities

The choice of modality of food delivery in school has considerable implications, both for program objectives and from the costs perspective. On the basis of the current data, in-school meals are approximately three times more costly than fortified biscuits. Furthermore, as shown in table 5.1, biscuits are more cost efficient with regard to energy and micronutrient delivery, offering potential advantages in contexts where micronutrient deficiencies in school-age children are widespread and the infrastructure and resources for school meal programs are constrained. However, biscuits fall far short of the overall nutritional benefits offered by a meal and do not substitute for a meal.

Additionally, the choice of school feeding modality is always going to be locally specific. The decisions made by Panama's school feeding program offer an example of such considerations. Food items in the Panama program include milk, fortified *crema* (evaporated milk and sugar), fortified biscuits, and lunch, with the cost of these different items varying substantially. Among the snack options (milk, crema, and biscuits), crema is least expensive as measured by cost per ration, per 1,000 kcal, and per 100 grams of protein (see table 5.2). Although milk costs twice as much, law in Panama states all schoolchildren have the right to a free daily serving of milk, legislation that appears to have "strong backing from the milk processing and packaging lobby in Panama" (World Bank 2000, annex 16, p. 4). So even though replacing milk with crema would improve the cost-effectiveness of the program, milk has been retained because it is protected by law.

**Table 5.1    Comparison of Average Annual Cost per Beneficiary, and per Nutrient Delivery for Fortified Biscuits and On-Site Meals, US$**

| Modality | Standardized cost per beneficiary per year | Cost per 100 kcals delivered | Cost per mg of iron delivered | Cost per 100 mcg of vitamin A delivered | Cost per 100 mcg of iodine delivered |
|---|---|---|---|---|---|
| On-site | 40 | 11 | 9 | 19 | 130 |
| Biscuits | 13 | 5 | 2 | 4 | 19 |

*Sources:* Galloway et al. forthcoming; Gelli et al. 2006.
*Note:* mcg = microgram; mg = milligram.

**Table 5.2    Comparison of Different Item Costs for a School Feeding Program in Panama, US$**

| Item | Cost per ration | Cost per 1,000 kcal | Cost per 100 grams of protein |
|---|---|---|---|
| Milk | 0.21 | 1.33 | 2.62 |
| Crema | 0.09 | 0.55 | 2.22 |
| Biscuit | 0.13 | 0.84 | 5.70 |
| Lunch | 0.13 | 0.20 | 0.80 |

*Source:* World Bank 2000.

## Trade-Offs in Targeting and Feeding Modalities

Table 5.3 summarizes the issues discussed in this chapter, and seeks to provide the school feeding policy maker with the key information for making informed choices. School feeding programs are context specific, and choices will ultimately depend upon balancing the key outcomes sought against the trade-offs and costs that will be incurred. One major deficit is the lack of reliable cost data. This is surprising given the popularity of school feeding programs. The current cost estimates fall in the lower range of those reported in earlier work by the World Bank, where the cost of programs providing food through schools standardized over 365 days and 1,000 kcals varied from US$19.35 to US$208.59 per recipient and average costs by region ranged from US$79 in Sub-Saharan Africa to US$91 in Asia (Horton 1992). More accurate estimates of costs are an important area for future research.

An even more important omission is a meaningful estimate of the cost efficiency of the different modalities and targeting approaches. For example, while it seems possible from the research that fortified biscuits have less impact on cognition than meals (see chapter 3), the scale of this difference is largely unknown. There is similar uncertainty about the extent to which meals or take-home rations are the better choice for encouraging enrollment. Research to estimate costs should specifically also seek to relate the costs to the scale of outcome. In particular, there are very few studies that compare meals and take-home rations in similar settings. The two that have gone farthest with this (that is, the Burkina Faso and Uganda studies; Alderman et al. 2008) suggest that both programs lead to similar improvements over having no program at all; thus, the choice of program types might hinge on the costs of delivery.

**Table 5.3  School Feeding Modalities, Outcomes, Trade-Offs, Costs, and Type of Food**

| | Meals | Snacks or high-energy biscuits | Take-home rations |
|---|---|---|---|
| **Expected benefits** | • May have significant educational benefits related to enrollment, attendance, dropout, educational achievement, and cognition.<br>• May reduce micronutrient deficiencies depending on the food basket and complementary interventions.<br>• Provide an immediate food transfer. | • Similar to meals in educational achievement and cognition, but perhaps lower benefits on enrollment and attendance.<br>• May reduce micronutrient deficiencies depending on the contents of the biscuit and complementary interventions.<br>• Provide an immediate food transfer. | • May have benefits on enrollment, attendance, and dropout (especially for girls and orphans and vulnerable children, if so targeted); emerging evidence for benefits for educational achievement.<br>• Provide an immediate food transfer. |
| **Advantages and trade-offs** | • From a safety net point of view, transfer value is limited to the amount of food the child eats at school.<br>• Food basket may be tailored to local tastes and cultural habits.<br>• Require community involvement and participation.<br>• Appropriate for full-day and boarding schools.<br>• Food basket more expensive than biscuits but cheaper than take home rations<br>• Costs may be contained by modifying the food basket (for example, using micronutrient powders). | • Useful to reach a wider number of children at a lower cost than on-site meals.<br>• Easier to serve early in the school day (important to address short-term hunger).<br>• Energy content insufficient for long school day schedules or boarding schools.<br>• Less infrastructure requirements (no cooking, limited storage, longer shelf life). Useful especially in urban or emergency settings.<br>• Because they are considered snacks, there is a reduced risk that the child will get less food at home because of substitution. | • From a safety net point of view, they function much like conditional cash transfers and are useful when no conditional cash transfer is in place.<br>• They can give higher transfer values than on-site meals or snacks.<br>• Traditionally targeted to certain groups of vulnerable children but could be distributed widely to reach particularly vulnerable households.<br>• Do not require cooking or storage.<br>• Require less community involvement but teacher time to monitor attendance and establish entitlements.<br>• Evidence that they also benefit preschool children. |

|  | | |
|---|---|---|
| • Require cooking facilities, storage at school, community involvement, and teacher monitoring. | • Less need for community or teacher involvement.<br>• The effect of snacks or biscuits on enrollment or attendance of children depends on the extent to which they are considered a meaningful incentive to children and their families. | |
| **Costs**[a] | • Average US$40 per child per year (Galloway et al. forthcoming) | • Average US$13 per child per year for high-energy biscuits (Gelli et al. 2006) | • US$52 per child per year, average of four WFP operations (Gelli, Al-Shaiba, and Espejo forthcoming) |
| **Type of food** | • Cereals: maize (whole or meal), wheat flour, bulgur wheat, sorghum, or rice<br>• Pulses: beans, lentils, peas<br>• Meat, fish, chicken<br>• Vegetable oil<br>• Sugar<br>• Salt | • Fortified blended foods such as corn-soya blend<br>• Fortified biscuits | • Vegetable oil<br>• Cereals (maize, millet, sorghum, rice)<br>• Beans |

Source: Authors.

Note: a. Actual costs of individual school feeding programs vary from costs presented. For advocacy purposes, WFP uses a general school feeding figure of US$0.25 per day and US$50 per child per year.

# CHAPTER 6

# Institutional and Procurement Arrangements

This chapter continues the theme of how the sustainability and effectiveness of school feeding programs can be optimized by evidence-based decisions about program design. The previous chapter examined how program objectives can be met through trade-offs between different targeting approaches and feeding modalities, and the attendant costs. Here we explore how institutional arrangements and procurement choices can respond to the specific country context, especially in relation to policy, resources, and capacity, the three main factors that emerged from the analysis of the key determinants of the transition process.

## Institutional Arrangements

In many low-income countries, school feeding programs are managed by external implementing partners, often as a program that runs in parallel with sectoral programs. An important consequence of this is that any transition to national ownership requires as a first step the institutionalization of school feeding within national and local-level structures.

Many case studies of countries that have transitioned to national ownership point to the fact that, independent of context, programs benefit from having a designated institution in charge of the program at the central level. In a majority of countries, this responsibility lies with the education sector, although some countries have chosen to create independent institutions, particularly where the program is seen as a political priority. In other cases, the program may be viewed as a multisectoral intervention, crucially linked with the education sector, but implemented with agriculture, health, or local government. The key factor that sows the seeds for transition is government leadership for the incorporation of the program within national policy.

Where the food comes from and who is responsible for its purchase determines to a great extent how a program is managed. A program that buys large quantities of food from national traders and distributes it across the country will need significant centralized capacity to plan requirements well in advance, coordinate national level tenders, and manage distribution. In contrast, if the food is bought close to the schools using a decentralized system, then the institutional arrangements can be lighter at the national level, but with significant support to local-level structures. Thus, the roles and responsibilities of the different parts of the institutional system depend largely on the procurement modality and sources of food.

### Central Management

The nationally centralized model places overall management responsibility at the national or state level and typically relies on contractors and traders for food procurement. While there is community contribution and participation, such as from school or community gardens and parent and teacher involvement in the daily activities of the program, the main financial and management ownership for the program rests with the government institutions. Irrespective of location, the institutional home for the program needs to have the trained staff and budgeted resources to plan and manage the program.

Some countries have successfully integrated the implementation of school feeding activities with school health interventions such as deworming and, consequently, clustered staff at the district level to deal with these issues. In others, school feeding activities are handled by officials from a relevant sector. In either case, the planning, monitoring, and managing of a school feeding program require capacity at the local level, and training and budget to match. This type of implementation model, however, is becoming less politically popular and there is an increasing trend to rely on school-based management systems for school feeding, as with other aspects of the education sector.

## *Decentralized Models of School Feeding*

A high-level consultation on school feeding in Ghana reported in 2007 that most African countries now use a decentralized, or bottom-up approach that relies heavily on local structures (NEPAD 2007). Decentralization allows greater room for creative, albeit informal, implementation that better responds to local needs and contexts, which in turn may foster local community involvement. Nigeria's decentralized, informal procurement system, for instance, allows each school management committee to purchase foodstuffs and develop menus that reflect local dietary patterns and traditions. Such services are better able to use locally adapted technologies, support coordinated community action, and promote partnerships.

A decentralized implementation model, while having these advantages, also raises certain important issues. Decentralization may result in uneven implementation. Ghana's school feeding program, although rolled out nationwide under high-level political leadership, shows differences at the regional, district, and school levels in administration structure, procurement practices, menu development, and meal preparation. This is also true in Brazil, India, and South Africa, where a diversity of practices can be observed at each implementation level (WFP 2009). Communities and schools with greater resources, political support, or local initiatives may have stronger programs, creating regional disparities or exacerbating existing inequalities. Communities and schools most in need of the benefits of school feeding may be left out.

The decentralized model places more responsibility on district and regional levels and draws on the strengths of existing community-based institutions, such as school management committees and village groups. In some areas of Ghana, food is procured by the District Commissioners, while in Nigeria and Thailand local school structures are responsible. Elsewhere, women's groups, school committees, and farmer-based organizations play a role. In all of these approaches the aim is to site decision making within the beneficiary community, and to enhance transparency and local accountability.

Context-specific approaches are especially important. For example, in urban areas with high population density, the management of the program could be organized with several large kitchens serving a large number of schools and children. In India, 15 kitchens in 6 states provide food to 5,700 schools and 960,000 students daily as part of the national Mid-Day Meal Program at a cost of US$28 per child per year. This approach might be less appropriate in a rural setting where schools are small and far apart from each other (Akshaya Patra Foundation 2008).

### Community-Sustained Programs

It is important to find the right balance between programs that count on community participation and ownership—a very positive factor in sustainability—and programs that seek to be largely funded by communities. There is a tendency to consider community-sustained programs as an option in reducing dependence on external assistance, but this places significant expectations on communities that they may not be able to fulfill. Indeed, there is anecdotal evidence from many low-income countries that communities introduce fees or in-kind contributions to support such programs, and by so doing erect barriers to education, particularly for girls and the poor.

Additionally, this type of program by definition can only be sustained in food-secure and generally better-off areas in a country and cannot serve the populations that are most in need. Similarly, this model is particularly susceptible to shocks (for example, rising food prices or drought) and may have problems regarding the type, quality, and regularity of meals distributed. Nevertheless, such programs may have a place in an overall national strategy, for example, by serving better-off communities, and case studies on community-sustained school feeding could help to gain a better understanding of good practice as well as possible pitfalls in this regard and of the extent to which communities can fund and sustain school feeding in different contexts.

In some cases, communities themselves establish school feeding programs independent of formal structures. And in many places, this is the only model implemented. Because it is already established, it could be an effective channel to distribute additional resources to communities. In Togo, for example, where there is no formal school feeding program, children are usually given a small allowance by their parents to buy meals prepared and sold by members of the community (the *mamans*). This system is relatively efficient but is becoming increasingly expensive because of the food price crisis. By the end of the 2007/08 school year, the cost of a basic meal (for example, 120 grams of rice with fish sauce) had increased by almost 50 percent. As a response to the food price crisis, the government is developing a food stamps program, using external funds to provide vouchers to children to buy lunch from the mamans.

In cases where the government has decided to place responsibility on the community for sustaining the school feeding program, specific support to communities could be put in place, for example, by linking agricultural programs to communities. Also, a solid policy framework would still be needed that recognizes the existence of this program and an institutional setup would be needed to determine guidelines, minimum standards, and support to the community. In certain cases, the government may wish to consider a mixed model of implementation, where a basic food basket would be provided by the state, which could then be complemented by the community. This way, the food supply of the program could be protected, and minimum nutritional and quality standards could be maintained.

## The Role of the Private Sector in School Feeding

The need for national policy on school feeding and an institutional framework to manage the program does not imply that implementation should only be done by the public sector. In many cases the private sector can play a very important role not only in the production of the food but also in the management and distribution functions of the program. There are examples, such as Chile, where national policy specifically outsources responsibility to the private sector for the majority of implementation functions. Equally, there are other countries that have a mix of public-private partnerships in implementation, for example, India, which has both state-administered programs and those supported by private sector organizations. At the local level, small and medium enterprises can also be involved in catering for the program, multiplying the effect on the local economy. The sections below describe the main procurement mechanisms for school feeding, which could be done by the state, by external organizations, by the private sector, or by a combination of two or more of these actors.

## Procurement

Procurement mechanisms are central to implementation. They depend on the availability of cash versus in-kind resources for the programs, and on the local food security situation. When cash resources are available, whether from donors or national sources, the procurement arrangements need to strike a balance between the cost efficiency of the procurement mechanisms that are chosen, the quality of the food, and the possible impact on local markets.

There are four main ways in which food is provided to school feeding programs:

- procurement outside of the country (international or regional)
- procurement within the country

- procurement local to the schools
- community-sustained.

The requirements, potential benefits, and trade-offs implicit in each approach are described in table 6.1. International procurement was the approach most commonly used by WFP and other development partners providing food aid support for school feeding in low-income countries. Procurement within country and local procurement are the most common approaches within national programs, and are now emerging as the more common approaches. In many cases, a combination of different procurement modalities is needed to achieve a maximum level of efficiency.

### *Accountability and Monitoring of Procurement*

As with other programs that involve substantial quantities of commodities and long-term contracts, there are opportunities for corrupt practices in procurement and contracting associated with school feeding programs. While it is usually recognized that procurement from outside the country—regional or international—requires systematic tendering and bidding processes, there may be less awareness that these are also necessary and appropriate for competitive procurement, even down to the district level. There is anecdotal evidence that procurement at the lower administrative levels may raise particular concerns because of the distance from the central monitoring processes. Bidding may not be appropriate or possible, however, in highly localized procurement from small-scale farmers, where instead a transparent process with broad community involvement and oversight may provide an effective alternative. This approach has proven effective in school-based management of budgets, provided that both inflows and expenditures are transparently shared within the beneficiary community. Procurement contracts for such components as transport, storage, and food preparation constitute another area where close monitoring and oversight are required, linked with strong tendering processes and transparency.

When governments or municipalities have a legal mandate for school feeding programs, there is often a legally specified composition for the food basket. This may provide an opportunity for special interest groups, for example, dairy producers or those packaging perishable products such as liquid milk, to benefit from preferential markets, especially if the selection of the composition is inadequately separated from potential political influence.

**Table 6.1  Requirements, Benefits, and Trade-Offs of Different Types of Procurement**

| Type of procurement | Requirements | Potential benefits | Risks and trade-offs |
|---|---|---|---|
| Procurement outside the country (regional or international) | • System of tenders in place<br>• Logistics capacity to move food internationally | • In food-insecure, landlocked countries it might be the only alternative<br>• Possible better prices than in national procurement | • Possible delays in arrival of food leading to breaks in the food pipeline<br>• Does not stimulate local production<br>• Food might not be what communities are used to eating |
| Procurement within the country | • System of national tenders in place<br>• Production capacity of the area is enough to cope with demand without affecting market prices<br>• Possible storage capacity at different points in country<br>• If done by the government, strong institutional structure and capacity at the central level, including a team of officers dedicated to planning, procurement, and logistics | • Potential for developing national production and processing capacity<br>• Wide choice in food basket options (fortified food, biscuits, blended food, other products not grown in the locality, and so forth)<br>• Potential to negotiate prices if buying in bulk and to protect against defaults<br>• Food can be moved from food-secure areas to schools in food-insecure areas | • Transportation and logistics might be expensive and cumbersome<br>• Storage capacity might not be there at national level |

*(continued)*

**Table 6.1 Requirements, Benefits, and Trade-Offs of Different Types of Procurement** *(Continued)*

| Type of procurement | Requirements | Potential benefits | Risks and trade-offs |
|---|---|---|---|
| Procurement local to the school | • Production capacity of the area is enough to cope with demand without affecting market prices<br>• Transparent system for district or regional tenders in place<br>• Quality control mechanisms in place | • Local agricultural production and economy may be stimulated<br>• Food basket may be culturally appropriate<br>• Transportation and storage costs may be lower as a result of shorter distances | • Local processing capacity might not be there to ensure proper fortification of food or production of specific foodstuffs like high-energy biscuits or corn-soya blend<br>• Quality control of the food might be difficult<br>• Risk of default on contracts may be high<br>• Vulnerability to volatile district and regional food prices in some areas<br>• Vulnerability to regional food insecurity, which might put food pipeline in danger<br>• May excessively burden local-level structures (districts, teachers, and communities) |
| Community-sustained school feeding | • In-kind or cash contributions from communities<br>• System works only in productive areas in countries | • Greater community ownership<br>• Better response to local needs and contexts<br>• Fosters local community involvement | • Does not necessarily channel additional resources into the community<br>• Does not work in animal grazing areas or extremely food insecure areas, which may need school feeding the most<br>• Economic shocks, like rising food prices, may affect the ability of communities to provide food for the program |

*Source:* Authors.

## The Multiplier Effect of Local Procurement

As discussed in chapter 4, local procurement is being actively evaluated by countries and development partners as a means to achieve sustainable school feeding programs, and at the same time to use the purchasing power of the program as a stimulus for the local agricultural economy. As such, local purchase of food for school feeding is seen as a force multiplier, benefiting children and the local economy at the same time. The following section explores the lessons learned on implementing local procurement in low-income countries, based on the limited experience to date.

There are few operational examples of local procurement programs in Africa, though several programs are being planned. Existing information from case studies illustrates that there are different ways of linking the school feeding program to local production. Some options include procuring foodstuffs from farmer cooperatives or associations, engaging with the private sector to produce fortified products for school feeding at a large scale, supporting local small and medium businesses to cater for the program, and encouraging school committees to buy the food requirements in local markets. In South Africa, for example, the school feeding program focuses on creating employment opportunities for women, encouraging them to form small businesses that provide for the school feeding program in a given area. In some regions in Ghana, resources are channeled to the school committee, which is responsible for buying, storing, and preparing the food in the school.

A recent study on locally sourced school feeding programs (WFP 2009) identified the potential value of the approach, but also a number of issues that need to be addressed in implementing this type of program.

School feeding must guarantee an uninterrupted supply of food that meets nutrition and health standards. The need to fortify food would add food processing as an additional step in the value chain. In Malawi, for example, a pilot project is supporting five community bakeries to manufacture and deliver fortified scones to schools. Another option is to add micronutrient powders to locally sourced food as necessary (see chapter 5). Attention must be paid to hygiene and food handling practices at the local level.

Procurement at local levels may be problematic because of high transaction costs, high risk of default, difficulties in meeting quality standards, and delays in delivery. At least in the initial stages, procurement at local levels should be combined with more traditional procurement mechanisms to protect the food pipeline.

The new market may also offer perverse incentives. If the demand for food from the school feeding program is significantly greater than the actual supply of food in the market, prices may temporarily increase, negatively affecting net buyers of food and further increasing their food insecurity until producers and traders adjust. Small-scale farmers may begin to cultivate more of the crop needed for the school feeding program to the detriment of other crops that had been cultivated, affecting crop diversity. To tackle these issues, systematic market and supply assessments should be done at different stages in the implementation of the program.

Based on the information from case studies and modeling exercises, the authors of the study (WFP2009) propose a three-phase process for implementing a locally sourced school feeding program. They project that costs will rise during the first phase (as a result of new procurement procedures and administrative costs of buying locally); peak during the second phase (because of added agricultural interventions in conjunction with the program); and finally, decrease during the third phase.

## School-Level Implementation Arrangements

School feeding programs that respond to community needs, are locally owned, and incorporate some form of parental or community contribution, whether cash payment or in-kind, for example, through donated food or labor, tend to be the strongest programs and the ones most likely to make a successful transition from donor assistance. Programs that build this component in from the beginning and consistently maintain it have the most success. Arrangements, however, have to be made to avoid increasing the cost of schooling to parents.

Schools normally put in place canteen or food management committees composed of representatives of parents, teachers, and students. The role of the committee is to act as an interface between the community and the school, manage the school feeding program, and ensure good utilization of the food in the school. Strong management committees ensure that teachers do not carry the entire burden of running the program. They should also ensure that children—especially girls—are not engaged in cooking, and that eating times are appropriately scheduled so they do not interfere with teaching.

There are very significant opportunity costs of using teachers to prepare food. Additional responsibilities for teachers, especially in the decentralized models of school feeding where teachers sometimes purchase the food, have negative implications for children's education. Field work in India shows that teachers in charge of the school feeding activities need an average of two to three hours every day away from teaching. While children's learning opportunities might be increased by providing them with food at school, children may also be disadvantaged if their teachers have fewer hours for classroom teaching as a result of their added responsibilities.

School gardens are often done in conjunction with school feeding and aim to provide a learning experience to children on sustainable agricultural production, the use of improved and locally appropriate technologies, and nutrition concepts. In practice, experience is variable, especially where teachers have limited experience with agriculture. Emphasis is normally put on diversification of food crops, fruits, vegetables, and weather-resistant varieties of several grains and staples. The products of the school garden can be used to complement the food provided in the school feeding program and enhance dietary diversity. School gardens, however, should not be expected to sustain the program, and care should be taken to ensure that the gardens do not detract from teaching and students' learning.

## Environmental Concerns at the School Level

There are significant environmental concerns that arise from school feeding operations, and all modalities may have associated negative impacts.

The preparation of in-school meals requires the use of fuel. In many situations where this occurs in the school or community this will involve the use of wood or charcoal from the adjacent area, contributing to deforestation. The construction of fuel-efficient stoves can significantly reduce fuel consumption and help minimize impact.

Challenges may arise from the management and disposal of packaging and wrapping, especially milk cartons and biscuit wrappings. Reusable sacks and cans are to be encouraged, and schools and communities can re-use or sell those empty food containers.

**Box 6.1**

## Case Studies: School Feeding Programs in Transition from Stage 1 to Stage 2
(for further details, see table 4.1)

*Sudan*

In 2008, a school feeding program in Sudan reached about 1.2 million children throughout the country with the objectives of increasing school attendance, particularly of girls, and relieving short-term hunger, while transferring resources to vulnerable households. Lack of food in the household is reportedly one of the main reasons for dropout, according to a baseline survey done by the Ministry of Education in 2008 (Sudan Ministry of General Education 2008). About two-thirds of the beneficiaries of the program are from South Sudan and Darfur.

*The benefits of the program.* The combination of conflict, large-scale population displacement, and poverty makes Sudan a complex environment in which to operate a school feeding program. The ongoing conflict in Darfur; the challenges confronting South Sudan after decades of civil war, including returning populations, limited infrastructure, and the need for the consolidation of governance; strained livelihoods; and economic dislocation in the East have left much of Sudan food insecure. A 2007 evaluation of school feeding in emergency situations reviewed the program and found that in areas affected by conflict, displaced children are attracted to school sooner when there is a school feeding program than when there is none, providing an important stabilizing effect and facilitating social cohesion. The evaluation also highlighted that the common meal provided in school provides an important psychosocial support to children affected by conflict (WFP 2007d).

*The challenges of implementing in a complex environment.* Despite these benefits, implementing school feeding in a fragile context is not without its challenges. The main issue is achieving a balance between the needs of vulnerable populations and the feasibility of operating the program in unstable areas. Some of the constraints include inaccessibility because of poor road networks, lack of partners able to manage the program in remote areas, lack of flexibility for adjustment of program modalities, poor school infrastructure and limited community capacity to manage the program, high costs resulting from complex logistical operations, and insecurity for implementing staff and beneficiaries.

The program is implemented under the Ministry of Education with support from WFP.

*(continued)*

**Box 6.1** *(Continued)*

*Haiti*

The government of Haiti's proposed approach toward school feeding is outlined in the National Strategy for Education for All. The strategy calls for reaching 30 percent of all schoolchildren, prioritizing schools in poor and marginalized areas. The service delivery model proposes to offer deworming and micronutrient fortification as components to feeding programs. Institutional strengthening of the National School Feeding Program (PNCS) is also featured. The school feeding component of the World Bank International Development Association-supported Education for All (EFA) project is executed by PNCS, which subcontracts with private firms and nongovernmental organizations to deliver the feeding programs to schools in select areas. The project reaches 45,000 children with these services, aiming to provide 1,000 kcal per child per day. The International Development Association support will also pilot a community-based school feeding program beginning in school year 2009/10, based on models in Guyana and Brazil. The WFP-supported school feeding program in Haiti reached 300,000 children in 2007.

*Nutritional security in Haiti: Enhancing existing mechanisms.* The government of Haiti, WFP, the World Bank, UNICEF, and the World Health Organization have been working together to improve the capacity and effectiveness of nutrition-related programs, with the view of safeguarding the nutritional security of Haiti's most vulnerable populations. The technical assistance project takes a two-pronged approach, focusing on quick wins and just-in-time advice to improve existing programs, and actions that, while focusing on nutrition, begin to lay the foundation for other qualitative improvements in Haiti's safety net.

The three thematic areas that the project focuses on are (1) knowledge and information, which includes activities such as mapping of service delivery, gathering data on growth monitoring, and carrying out a national survey on children's nutritional health; (2) strengthening nutritional security programs, which includes adding nutrition and family health elements to existing school feeding programs, and piloting new approaches to reduce malnutrition, focusing on community participation; and (3) building constituency and institutions for nutritional security.

# CHAPTER 7

# How to Design and Update School Feeding Programs

Previous chapters highlight the need to improve the design of new school feeding programs and to revisit existing programs with a view toward sowing the seeds for sustainability and effectiveness. This chapter presents a compilation of existing tools and two new tools to assist program designers and policy makers.

The available tools tend to concentrate on the design and implementation of programs, but typically lack guidance on how to assess and put in place the key factors that lead to sustainability. In particular, there is a need for guidance on how to analyze the policy framework in a given country, the financial capacity and funding alternatives for the program, and the institutional arrangements and implementation capacity. There is also a need to update existing guidance on the trade-offs in choosing among the different modalities, the options for the food basket, the relative costs, and the expanded range of procurement options. In response to this need, this section describes an updated checklist (presented in detail in appendix 3) as a tool to guide the design of new school feeding programs.

Just as there is a need for clear guidance on how to design effective and sustainable programs from the start, there is also a growing recognition of the need to revisit and update existing programs. The analysis of the El Salvador case history (see appendix 1) shows that the transition process involved a significant investment of time and resources in changing over from one strategy to another. A growing number of countries have begun to use national consultations on school feeding as the basis for systematic strategic and practical dialogue among government and stakeholders, and as a starting point for the transition process. In this section we present a framework (described in detail in appendix 4) as a tool to facilitate the redesign of existing school feeding programs and to provide a common base for all stakeholders involved in the program.

A conclusion of these analyses is that the currently available tools to design school feeding need to be updated in light of new findings and knowledge on the topic.

## Checklist to Design and Implement New School Feeding Programs

Appendix 3 provides a checklist to design new school feeding programs. The tool suggests a step-by-step process, including the following main stages:

- *Problem analysis* includes assessments to determine the operational context and the possible role and need for school feeding. It also details a feasibility assessment and an analysis of government policies related to school feeding.
- *Definition of objectives* clarifies the program's objectives and the expected outcomes based on the assessment and problem analysis results.
- *Targeting* identifies the relevant groups and target areas, based on assessment results.
- *Rations composition and food distribution modality* details the need to select the type of food, the type of rations, and modalities that are in line with program objectives, practical aspects, and costs.
- *Management and implementation arrangements* include school-level management arrangements, monitoring and evaluation systems, coordination, and complementary activities.
- *Risk management and contingency planning* identifies possible risks to program implementation and strategies to mitigate them.
- *Costing and budgeting* includes a breakdown of costs by set-up costs and continuing costs and possible funding sources.

## Checklist to Update Existing School Feeding Programs

Recent interest in school feeding has led to national discussions in many countries. Governments have held national consultations or workshops around the issue as a first step toward including the program in national policy. There is a growing need for a framework to guide these types of conversations among stakeholders and partners and to provide a systematic way of thinking about school feeding and its implications at the national and subnational levels.

Appendix 4 presents a tool to revisit school feeding programs in light of new thinking and research. It is meant to be an assessment framework that can be used by the government or by other partners to assess the quality and potential for sustainability of an existing school feeding program. The tool is meant to provide a road map for a smooth transition of a school feeding program to the government and therefore serve as the basis for a transition strategy. It also provides a framework within which the government and partners can collectively discuss, analyze, and take action on school feeding around a set of common objectives. As such, it can enhance national ownership, facilitate dialogue between partners and the government, guide action planning and capacity development strategies, and help to focus resources on specific priority areas.

To date, this tool has been used in Afghanistan, Haiti, Malawi, and Pakistan as the basis for national workshops on school feeding. The results of the workshops have been action plans to improve the existing programs and coordinate actions among different stakeholders. It was used in Tanzania as the basis for the redesign of the school feeding program and in El Salvador as the framework for a transition case study (featured in appendix 1).

The tool has the following five components of school feeding and 20 indicators or benchmarks of good practice:

1. *Strong policy frameworks*
   - The national-level poverty reduction strategy or equivalent national strategy identifies school feeding as an education intervention, a social protection intervention, or both.
   - The sectoral policies and strategies identify school feeding as an education or social protection intervention (education sector plan, social protection policy).
   - There is a specific strategy related to school feeding or school health and nutrition that specifies the objectives, rationale, scope, design, and funding of the program.

2. *Strong institutional structure and coordination*
   - There is a national institution mandated with the implementation of school feeding.

- There is a specific unit in charge of the overall management of school feeding within the lead institution at the central level and that unit has sufficient staff, resources, and knowledge.
- There is an intersectoral coordination mechanism in place that is operational and involves all stakeholders and partners of the institution.
- There are adequate staff and resources for oversight at the regional level.
- There are adequate staff and resources for design and implementation at the district level.
- There are adequate staff, resources, and infrastructure for implementation at school level.

3. *Stable funding and planning*
   - School feeding is institutionalized within the national planning and budgeting process.
   - There is a budget line for school feeding and national funds from the government or from donors that cover the needs of the program regularly.

4. *Sound program design and implementation*
   - The program has appropriate objectives corresponding to the context and the policy framework.
   - Program design identifies appropriate target groups and targeting criteria corresponding to the objectives of the program and the context.
   - Program has appropriate food modalities and food basket corresponding to the context, objectives, local habits and tastes, availability of local food, and nutritional content requirements (demand-side considerations).
   - Procurement and logistics arrangements are based on procuring as locally as possible as often as possible taking into account the costs, the capacities of implementing parties, the production capacity in the country, the quality of the food, and the stability of the pipeline (supply and procurement considerations).
   - There is appropriate calibration of demand and supply, establishing what percentage of food demanded by the program can be sourced locally.
   - There is a monitoring and evaluation system in place and functioning that forms part of the structures of the lead institution and is used for implementation and feedback.

5. *Strong community participation and ownership (teachers, parents, children)*
   - The community has been involved in the design of the program.
   - The community is involved in the implementation of the program.
   - The community contributes (to the extent possible) resources (cash, in-kind) to the program.

## A Designer's Toolkit

Table 7.1 provides a selective list of available tools to design programs, from the initial assessment stage to the actual design of the program. Wherever possible, the list includes the URL where the tool can be found. All tools can be obtained by contacting WFP directly (wfpinfo@wfp.org).

**Table 7.1    Tools Available for School Feeding Design and Implementation**

| Name of tool | Description |
|---|---|
| **Assessment tools** | |
| Comprehensive Food Security and Vulnerability Analysis | In-depth assessments that provide information on food insecurity, the risks to livelihoods, and emerging food security problems. *Useful for situation analysis, targeting, risk mitigation plans* |
| Purchase for Progress Assessments | Provide information on national agricultural production, impediments to small farmer agricultural productivity, capacity of small farmer associations, factors affecting small farmer access to markets. *Useful for food basket design, food procurement strategies, risk mitigation plans for food procurement* |
| High Food Prices Assessments | Provide information on food prices in the region and in the country, and effects of high food prices on food insecurity, livelihoods, education, and nutrition. *Useful for problem analysis, program design* |
| **Design and implementation tools** | |
| School Feeding Handbook | Provides details on program design and implementation, including food basket considerations, targeting, community arrangements, monitoring and evaluation, complementary interventions. *Under revision; new version will be released in 2009* |

*(continued)*

**Table 7.1    Tools Available for School Feeding Design and Implementation**
*(Continued)*

| Name of tool | Description |
| --- | --- |
| School Feeding Redesign and Assessment Tool | A comprehensive list of indicators and targets to assess the quality of a school feeding program, featured in appendix 4. One-, two-, or three-day workshop materials based on the tool are also available. Training for facilitators of the workshops is under preparation. |
| School Feeding Targeting Guidelines | Provides guidance on geographic and school-level targeting of school feeding programs in stable and emergency and recovery contexts. *Under revision; new version will be released in 2009* |
| Emergency School Feeding Guidelines | Specific guidance on programming in emergencies. *Under revision; new version to be released in 2009* |
| Food Basket Calculator | Excel program that calculates the nutritional value of various food commodities. Specifies kcal, vitamins, minerals, and compares to required daily allowance. |
| Checklist for the use of milk in school feeding programs | Describes a range of practical issues to be considered when assessing the use of milk for a school feeding program. |
| WFP school feeding program documents | Specify the design and implementation arrangements for WFP's school feeding program in a country. http://www.wfp.org/operations/list |
| Food for Education Works | Consolidates the different analyses of the monitoring and evaluation data collected by WFP between 2002 and 2006 to strengthen the knowledge base and learning components of its school feeding programs. http://www.schoolsandhealth .org/sites/ffe/Key%20 Information/Food% 20for%20Education%20Works%202006.pdf |
| WFP Home-Grown School Feeding | Provides a framework for action on home-grown school feeding. |
| FAO Nutrition Education in Primary Schools | Provides planning guidance for developing nutrition curricula. http://www.fao.org/docrep/ 009/a0333e/a0333e00.htm |
| FAO Setting up and Running a School Garden | Assists teachers, parents, and communities in the design or improvement of school gardens. http://www.fao.org/docrep/009/a0218e/ A0218E00.htm |

**Table 7.1    Tools Available for School Feeding Design and Implementation**
*(Continued)*

| Name of tool | Description |
|---|---|
| Getting Started: OVC Food Assistance Programming | Defines terms such as OVC; provides project cycle guidance for OVC programming, from needs assessment, targeting, partnerships, through monitoring and evaluation.<br>*Useful for cash and food transfers programming* |
| Social Protection for Vulnerable Children in the Context of HIV and AIDS: Moving Towards a More Integrated Vision | Defines what is new about social protection and why it is so important in the context of HIV and AIDS. School feeding is mentioned as one of the social protection mechanisms that can be preventive, protective, promotional, and transformative. www.crin.org/docs/Social%20Protection,%20Greenblot.pdf |
| Social Protection in the Era of HIV and AIDS: Examining the Role of Food-Based Interventions | Defines terms such as social protection and social safety nets from different perspectives; examines the role of food-based interventions in support of orphans and vulnerable children in the context of HIV. http://www.wfp.org/sites/default/files/Social_Protection_in_the_Era_of_HIV_and_AIDS_EN.pdf |
| Food Assistance Programming in the Context of HIV | Provides comprehensive guidance on food assistance programming in the context of HIV. School feeding is approached from the perspective of education, social safety nets, and livelihood. http://www.fantaproject.org/publications/fapch.shtml |
| INEE Minimum Standards for Education in Emergencies, Chronic Crises, and Early Reconstruction | Contains guidance for design and implementation of school feeding as part of emergency education programs. Minimum standards handbook and toolkit include school feeding program checklist and guidelines. http://www.ineesite.org/toolkit/ |

*Source:* Authors.
*Note:* INEE = Inter-agency Network of Educatión in Emergencies; OVC = Orphans and vulnerable children.

## Additional Sources of Useful Information

- www.wfp.org/food_aid/school_feeding (information on WFP's approach to school feeding, school feeding action, work with partners, documents, latest news)
- www.wfp.org/country_brief (information on WFP operations, including school feeding, by country)

- www.schoolsandhealth.org (resources, documents, country information, news, and events about school feeding and other school health and nutrition programs)
- www.unesco.org/education/fresh (toolkits for different types of school health and nutrition interventions, including school feeding)
- www.gcnf.org (Web site of the Global Child Nutrition Foundation, which supports developing countries in starting or expanding school feeding programs)
- www.sign-schoolfeeding.org (information on the Ghana Home-Grown School Feeding Program and documents on the Dutch government's support of the program)
- www.worldbank.org/education/schoolhealth (information on World Bank operations and knowledge management for school health and nutrition)
- www.worldbank.org/safetynets (information on World Bank operations in social protection and safety nets)

---

**Box 7.1**

## World Food Programme Support for School Feeding

WFP supports school feeding programs in 70 countries reaching 20 million children each year, typically handling the procurement and logistics of food. In each case WFP works with governments to ensure that school feeding is complementary to basic education and does not disrupt the educational system. Communities and parents play an important role in managing the programs at school level. The level of involvement of the government varies depending on the situation. In least developed countries and in emergency and fragile environments,

**WFP School Feeding**
**Key Figures – 2007**

**Beneficiaries:** 19.3 million

**Gender:** 48% were girls

**By region**
  Latin America: 8.7%
  Middle East and Central Asia: 3.4%
  South and South-East Asia: 35.8%
  Sub-Saharan Africa: 51.8%, of which
    Eastern and Central Africa: 21.3%
    Southern Africa: 9.7%
    The Sudan: 4.1%
    West Africa: 16.7%

**By modality**
  School meals: 90.4%
  Only take-home rations: 9.6%

**Food distribution:** 535,000 metric tons

**Estimated expenditures:** US$357 million

*(continued)*

**Box 7.1** *(Continued)*

WFP takes on the bulk of the responsibility to fund and manage the program. In more stable development situations, when school feeding is a government priority, governments progressively fund and manage the programs themselves, leading to an eventual phasing out of external assistance. As the government slowly takes on more financial and management responsibility, WFP's role changes, from purchasing and delivering the food to providing policy advice and technical assistance.

WFP is the largest international supporter of school feeding programs in low-income countries, valued at over US$357 million. In 2007, the organization spent US$612 million buying food for all purposes in 69 developing countries. In 2008, the value of WFP food commodities procured in developing countries was $882 million.

WFP is piloting a series of efforts to purchase some of the food for its programs locally from small-scale farmers through the Purchase for Progress program. By integrating its purchasing power with the technical contributions of other partners to connect small-scale and low-income farmers to markets, WFP envisions that within five years, participating low-income farmers will realize higher annual farming income as a direct result of sales of commodities to WFP. Also envisioned is that best practices in pro-smallholder local food procurement and agricultural market development for low-income farmers will have been identified and mainstreamed in WFP's policies and program practices. Lessons will also be shared with national governments and other public and private sector actors in the agricultural sector.

By redesigning food procurement practices, WFP can play an active role in connecting farmers to markets by transferring its know-how and tools to local producers to ensure that they are more competitive in the agricultural marketplace, including the market created by WFP. Activities will be piloted in at least the following countries over the next five years: Afghanistan, Burkina Faso, Democratic Republic of Congo, Ethiopia, Guatemala, Kenya, the Lao People's Democratic Republic, Liberia, Malawi, Mali, Mozambique, Nicaragua, Rwanda, Sierra Leone, Sudan, Tanzania, Uganda, and Zambia. In these and other countries, school feeding programs are being used as a source of demand for new procurement models. To do this, WFP is analyzing the food basket for school feeding and ensuring that it is based on locally available nutritious foods, wherever possible, and that the supply of food for school feeding programs is carefully calibrated, factoring in national production capacity and building deliberate links to small farmers.

**Box 7.2**

## Case Study: School Feeding Program in Transition from Stage 3 to Stage 4
(for further details, see table 4.1)

### Kenya

WFP has provided school meals to children in Kenya for the last 28 years. In 2008, school meals were provided to about 1,210,000 children in more than 3,800 schools in vulnerable areas within 63 districts and 6 Nairobi slums. The main objective of the program is to increase school enrollment and attendance. The targeted districts have the lowest school enrollment and attendance rates, as well as gender ratios, in the country compared with national averages, mainly as the result of cultural values, the poor state of school facilities, poverty, and hunger.

*Increasing government financial allocations.* Over the past years the government of Kenya has started allocating resources to the program through in-kind transfers of food that is locally produced. Management responsibilities are also being gradually transferred. The government receives external assistance for purchasing and providing the food for the program, while the government itself is responsible for food distribution from the warehouses to the assisted schools. The full cost of running the school feeding program in Kenya, including community contributions, was estimated at US$28 per child per year.

A range of contributions are also made by parents and other community members in each assisted school. The school management committee generally manages the program and agrees on fees that will be charged to each child in the school to support school feeding. If parents cannot afford to pay in cash, they provide in-kind contributions or services. The school levies charged for each child in Kenya are in the range of 100 to 300 Kenya shillings (US$1.38 to US$4.17) per child per year for rural and urban schools, respectively.

Recently the government of Kenya launched a Home-Grown School Feeding Programme, aimed at feeding some 550,000 schoolchildren previously fed by WFP, starting in the first term of 2009. An initial US$6 million was allocated by the government for the 2008/09 fiscal year for the program. A targeting exercise identified 28 marginal agricultural districts with access to markets for the new program. The cash is transferred directly to schools for local purchase of cereals, pulses, and oil.

# CHAPTER 8

# Key Findings and Research Agenda

The previous chapters examine the evidence base for school feeding programs with the overall objective of better understanding how to develop and implement effective school feeding programs in two contexts: (1) a productive safety net, as part of the response to the social shocks of the current global crises; and (2) a fiscally sustainable investment in human capital, as part of long-term global efforts to achieve Education for All and provide social protection to the poor.

## Key Findings of the Analyses

Here we summarize the key findings of the main analyses.

### The Current Global Coverage of School Feeding Programs

- Every country (for which we have data) is in some way and at some scale seeking to provide food to its schoolchildren.
- Comprehensive school feeding is near universal in those high- and middle-income countries that can afford the programs and for which we have data.
- Countries with the greatest need are those where the school feeding programs are currently least adequate.

The near universality of school feeding, and the inadequacy of programs where the need is greatest, suggest an important opportunity for development partners to assist governments to roll out safety nets in response to the current global crises, and to sow the seeds for longer-term investment in human capital and social protection.

### The Benefits of School Feeding Programs

- The primary drivers for increased support for school feeding are the benefits for social protection and for education.
- The social safety net roles of school feeding programs include an immediate response to social shocks as well as social protection over the longer term.
- School feeding can benefit education through enrollment, attendance, cognition, and educational achievement, although the scale of benefit and the evidence of effect vary with feeding modality.
- Well-designed school feeding programs that include micronutrient fortification and deworming can provide nutritional benefits and should be designed to complement and not compete with nutrition programs for younger children, which remain a clear priority for targeting malnutrition overall.

The focus on social protection and education benefits suggests a need for these sectors to be more systematically engaged in the development of school feeding programs, including research, design, and the policy dialogue.

### The Sustainability of School Feeding Programs

- Programs in low-income countries exhibit large variation in cost, with concomitant opportunities for cost containment.
- As countries grow economically from low to middle income, the cost of school feeding declines substantially relative to the cost of education, which argues for a particular focus on supporting programs in countries before they make that transformation.
- The main preconditions for the transition to sustainable national programs are mainstreaming school feeding in national policies and plans, especially education sector plans; national financing; and national implementation capacity.
- A key message is the importance of designing long-term sustainability into programs from their inception, and of revisiting programs as they

evolve. Countries benefit from having a clear understanding of the duration of donor assistance, a systematic strategy to strengthen institutional capacity, and a concrete plan for transition to national ownership with timeframes and milestones of the process.

Further benefits might accrue from better alignment of support for school feeding with the processes already established to harmonize development cooperation in the education sector, notably the Education for All-Fast Track Initiative.

### Trade-Offs in the Design of School Feeding Programs

- There are real differences in costs and benefits among the available modalities, and there are significant differences in the appropriateness of the different modalities to local capacity and contexts.
- Given a finite budget, targeting is essential to ensure that programs provide the most benefit to the intended beneficiaries, as well as maximize benefits and contain costs.
- There are significant and avoidable opportunity costs of using teachers to prepare food, and significant and avoidable environmental concerns that arise from school feeding operations, especially relating to cooking fuel and packaging.
- The participation of children and communities is a positive determinant factor in the sustainability of a program, but careful program design is required to avoid exploitation and negative implications for education.

Designing effective programs requires an evidence base that allows careful trade-offs among targeting approaches, feeding modalities, and costs. There is a particular need for better data on the cost-effectiveness of the available approaches and modalities.

### Institutional and Procurement Arrangements That Are Locally Appropriate and Ease the Transition to National Ownership

- Institutional arrangements and procurement choices should respond to the specific country context, especially in relation to policy, resources, and capacity.
- The management of school feeding programs has become increasingly decentralized, mirroring the trend in the education sector toward school-based management.

- Case studies of programs that have transitioned to sustainable national ownership show that programs benefit from having a designated national institution, usually the education sector, and appropriate capacity for implementation at subnational levels.
- Whereas national ownership appears to be a critical factor in transitioning to sustainability, many different approaches to implementation—including public sector, private sector, and public-private partnerships—appear to be effective.
- The roles and responsibilities of the institutional system depend largely on the procurement modality and sources of food. Within national programs, the two most common approaches are procurement within the country and local procurement, and these are now emerging as the most common approaches overall.
- Local procurement is being actively evaluated by countries as a means to achieve sustainable school feeding programs and at the same time stimulate the local agricultural economy by using the purchasing power of the program.
- Community-sustained programs are rarely an effective transition option for low-income countries because they introduce community costs that may be a barrier to education, especially for poor children and girls, and can only be sustained in food-secure areas.

The primary challenge in this area is how to build sustainability into programs from the outset. Case studies of countries that have transitioned to national ownership appear to provide useful guidance to other countries seeking to follow the same route, but there is also a need for assessment of new promising practices, especially the local purchase of food as a force multiplier, benefiting children and the local economy at the same time.

## Research Agenda

Here we list some of the key areas for research that were identified during the preparation of this book.

*A database on school feeding programs that describes the coverage and functioning of programs globally.* The most complete database currently available is that maintained by WFP for its own programs, but it focuses on low-income countries and does not provide information on programs implemented wholly by governments or by other agencies. It is not currently possible to estimate, for example, the global population served by school feeding programs, the gaps in coverage, the costs of different programs, the regularity of program functioning, or the popularity of different modalities.

***Assessment of the relative merits of school feeding versus other social safety net instruments.*** There is a concern that much of the data available may have limited external validity and there is a particular need for studies to explore the performance of social safety net instruments in low-income settings in Africa. Other safety net options, especially conditional cash transfer programs, tend to be small and rare in such settings, and school feeding programs are often part of a very limited choice of immediately available social protection instruments. Planning for the future requires a better understanding of the effectiveness of school feeding versus other safety net instruments.

***Impact studies that assess the education benefits of different designs of school feeding programs.*** There is a general need for large-scale, randomized trials that seek to provide reliable evidence of the impact of school feeding on education outcomes. Studies of all modalities are needed. There is a particular paucity of studies examining the relationship between education outcomes and (1) fortified biscuits and other fortified foods—most of the current evidence for the benefits of fortification is extrapolated from studies of supplementation—and (2) take-home rations. Impact studies should also assess the different institutional arrangements and their impact on benefits.

***Impact studies that assess the potential nutritional contribution of different designs of school feeding programs.*** This remains one of the most controversial areas of school feeding program design, not least because the obvious nutritional priority is younger children. More operational studies are required along the lines of the joint initiative by the government of Haiti, WFP, WHO, UNICEF, and the World Bank, which is exploring how to improve the capacity and effectiveness of nutrition-related programs, for example, by adding nutrition and family health elements to existing school feeding programs. Similarly, there is a need to address whether the nutritional benefits of school feeding programs for young children are comparable in cost-effectiveness with direct interventions targeted specifically at young children.

*Systematic estimates of the cost of the different school feeding modalities, and of the determinants of the considerable cost variation among countries.* The apparent variation in costs among low-income countries implies that there is considerable opportunity for cost containment, provided that the drivers of costs are better understood. The relevance of the modality is an important issue, and there is a particular lack of information on fortified biscuits (no data for Africa) and for take-home rations.

*The comparative cost-effectiveness and the relative benefits of different modalities of school feeding.* School feeding programs are context specific, and choices will ultimately depend upon balancing the key outcomes sought against the trade-offs and costs that will be incurred. This requires meaningful estimates of the cost efficiency of the different modalities as measured by outcomes. For example, while it seems probable from the research that some modalities may have less impact than others (for example, fortified biscuits versus meals), the scale of this difference is largely unknown.

*Case studies of countries that have successfully transitioned to sustainable programs.* The situation in specific countries is often complex, particularly where different school feeding models may exist in parallel in a country, and may vary from year to year. Progression from one model to the next may not be linear, especially where social shocks may reverse historical gains. Case studies could provide guidance on the transition process and help define the key elements of a successful transition strategy. These should also include information on how countries manage to finance these programs and how costs are borne within the country. The case studies should include the full range of options that have been explored, including the roles of the public sector, private-public partnerships, and the private sector; faith-based and other civil society organizations; and community-sustained programs.

*The capacity of local procurement schemes to provide additional economic and social benefits, and to contribute to sustainability by enhancing the cost-effectiveness of the operations.* Evidence indicates that local purchase schemes yield significant benefits in high- and middle-income countries. There is a need to support and add to the ongoing studies of the potential benefits of local procurement in Africa, which would include comparing the cost-effectiveness of local procurement versus other procurement options.

***Development of new technical guidance and knowledge management tools to support the design of school feeding programs.*** Existing tools to assist the design of school feeding programs need to be updated in light of new findings and knowledge on the topic, especially to include guidance on how to assess and put in place the key factors for sustainability.

# School Feeding in El Salvador: Preliminary Findings of a Case Study of the Transition

In 2008, the school feeding program in El Salvador became wholly owned and implemented by the government after 23 years of reliance on implementation partnerships, principally with the World Food Programme (WFP). The program started during the country's internal crisis in 1984, planning to reach 200,000 students from preschool through grade six in rural areas. In 1997, five years after the signing of the peace accords, the government began to take over program management responsibilities while WFP withdrew from departments no longer classified as among the most food insecure.

Currently, the government receives external support from WFP for technical assistance, logistics, and procurement through a trust fund that was established in 2008. Through this agreement, WFP is piloting procurement innovations under its corporate Purchase for Progress initiative, which aims to link local procurement with the school feeding program.

---

The preliminary findings presented here are reproduced with permission. The final version of this case study is being published elsewhere by Carmen Burbano, Aulo Gelli, and others.

## Documenting the Transition

In 2009, the government of El Salvador and WFP decided to carry out a study of the evolution of the school feeding program in El Salvador from 1984 to 2008 to document the process of transition to a nationally led program.

### *Objectives of the Study*

The study seeks to determine the critical factors and lessons learned from the transition experience, with the following specific objectives:

- To analyze the different steps or actions taken by government and partners that facilitated the transition toward a nationally owned program
- To identify best practices that might be replicated by other countries
- To identify lessons learned that might be taken into consideration by other countries.

### *Methodology*

The study covers school feeding activities from 1984 to 2008. It was done primarily through literature review and targeted interviews with the government and partners. Findings depended on the availability of historical information. There is a general gap in information from 1984 to 1992. Data from 1992 through early 2009 are fairly consistent, although there are some discrepancies between government and WFP sources. Here we present a preliminary analysis with the information available. The findings should be interpreted as a work in progress because more information will be collected in the future.

The study was structured around two simple questions:

1. Where are we now? To establish the current status and achievements of the program.
2. How did we get here? To identify the series of actions taken that led to that result.

Both questions were answered using the following framework to analyze the operational characteristics.

| Category | Where are we now? | How did we get here? |
|---|---|---|
| Policy frameworks | School feeding in the poverty reduction strategy, in sectoral policies, as a specific policy | How has the policy direction changed over time? What did WFP and partners do to influence that? What challenges were encountered? How were they solved? |
| Institutional frameworks | Current institutional responsibility, capacity of school feeding unit within the government, coordination mechanisms, capacity at decentralized structures | How has the institutional capacity evolved with time? How was it strengthened? What challenges were encountered? How were they solved? |
| Financial framework | Current school feeding within the national planning process, funding sources, possible funding gaps | How has the transition between WFP and government funding happened? How was the program funded? What arrangements did the government make? What did WFP do to help in this process? What challenges were encountered? How were they solved? |
| Program design | Current objectives, targeting, target groups, food basket | Have the objectives or target groups changed over time? Has the food basket changed or been modified to locally grown food? How? |
| Program implementation | Current procurement and logistics arrangements, amounts procured locally and regionally, calibration of demand and supply, monitoring and evaluation, complementary activities | How have procurement and logistics been handled over time? What are the main challenges? Successes? M&E successes and challenges? Deworming and other activities? |
| School-level arrangements and infrastructure | Current community role in design, implementation, monitoring. Participation and planning processes, priority setting. | How has the role of the community changed over time? How was it strengthened? Challenges? Successes? |

## Where Are We Now? The Current Status of School Feeding in El Salvador

The school feeding program in El Salvador annually reaches around 870,000 children, ages 5 to 15 years, in all rural and low-income urban areas. It is implemented as a social development program with the objectives of meeting the immediate food requirements of children, increasing enrollment and retention and reducing absenteeism, and improving the health habits of assisted children. School feeding also has a social protection role in the country, implicitly transferring resources to poor households. In fact, in 2008, the program was expanded to assist households affected by the rise in food prices.

School feeding in El Salvador has benefited from the support of several high-level political champions who have advocated the program's expansion and helped to ensure its sustainability. Currently, school feeding is the cornerstone of the country's multisectoral development program centered on children and youth called Escuela Saludable (Healthy Schools).

Public officials seem to agree that it would be politically very damaging to remove or even downscale the program given that public demand for school feeding is very high. School feeding has been the flagship program of the last two presidential campaigns, signaling its political sustainability.

This section explores the characteristics of the program on five levels: (1) policy framework, (2) institutional framework, (3) financial framework, (4) design and implementation, and (5) school-level arrangements and infrastructure. It also presents the main strengths and challenges of the program today and discusses some of the issues that the Ministry of Education is dealing with as it moves forward with the program.

### The National Policy Framework

Widespread commitment to the program is reflected in the country's policy and financial framework. School feeding is part of a wider multisectoral school health and nutrition initiative, called Escuela Saludable, managed by a division in charge of flagship social programs, which is attached to the President's Office, led by the First Lady. The program is also in the National Education Sector Plan, in the National Government Plan, and most important, in the operational plans of the Ministry of Education, which determines the budgetary requirements of the program.

According to government officials, one of the most important factors for the sustainability of the program is whether there is political and financial commitment to the program. In the case of El Salvador, commitment exists at the presidential and ministerial levels and there is a budget line for the program in the national budget.

### The Institutional Framework

As mentioned above, the program is part of the multisectoral initiative managed by a division attached to the President's Office. But the responsibility to design, manage, and implement the program lies with the Ministry of Education. A unit within the ministry that manages programs that are considered to be complementary to the provision of basic education (for example, life skills, health and nutrition, school feeding) is responsible for day-to-day activities. The unit has a director and 10 government officials assigned full time to the program, and an operational budget.

Oversight and coordination for Escuela Saludable are managed through a National Steering Committee chaired by the First Lady. Members include the Ministers of Education, Health, Agriculture, and Public Works. There is also a Technical Working Group in charge of following up decisions made by the Steering Committee.

El Salvador has 14 departments and in each there is a multisectoral team in charge of the program that manages activities at the local level. At the municipal level there are also staff and capacity for storage and distribution of food. At the school level, a school feeding committee headed by the director of the school and composed of parents and teachers oversees the daily implementation of the program.

### The Financial Framework

The program is currently financed exclusively with government funds. The majority of the program's requirements are covered through regular funds, following a 2005 decision by the Legislative Assembly to establish a budget line for school feeding. The rest of the requirements are covered through a trust fund that was established in 1999 with the proceeds from the privatization of the national telecommunications company. A national law requires that the interest generated by this fund be allocated to social programs, including school feeding. In 2008, the trust fund provided around US$3 million for school feeding. School feeding is embedded in the Ministry of Education's annual budget. The budget for school feeding in 2009 is US$17 million.

### Program Design and Implementation

The program currently provides a standardized on-site meal to more than 870,000 children. The meal provides about 26 percent and 20 percent of daily requirements for calories and protein, respectively. The food basket consists of rice, oil, fortified drink, beans, milk, and sugar.

Geographical targeting was done through two targeting studies using information from the Ministry of Education and two nutrition assessments done with the support of WFP. The program is targeted to children from 5 to 15 years old (preprimary, primary, and the first three grades of secondary) in all public schools in rural and low-income urban areas of the country. It is implemented in all 14 departments.

The ministry has a monitoring and evaluation system, managed at the central level. The system triangulates information from the overall coordinating unit in the President's Office, the Ministry of Education, and WFP. Information is collected at the input and output levels for assisted schools.

Although the government has fully taken over the management and financial responsibilities of the program, the Ministry of Education relies on external support for technical assistance to improve the efficiency of school feeding. Under a new agreement signed between the ministry and WFP in 2008, WFP assists the government with procurement and logistics for school feeding, and will undertake a study to redesign the food basket, training and sensitization at the local level, a review of the targeting procedures, and the establishment of a strategic food reserve for the program. These activities are done with national resources.

By leveraging its experience in food procurement in the region, WFP has been able to increase the efficiency of the procurement process. In 2008, WFP was able to buy all the food requirements of the program with less money than planned, generating savings for the government of about US$3 million. Savings were then used to expand coverage of the program and increase the food basket. Procurement is done nationally and regionally because there are seasonal food deficit periods in the country. There are plans to explore local purchase mechanisms under WFP's new Purchase for Progress initiative.

### School-Level Arrangements and Infrastructure

Food deliveries are done three times per year, and deposited in government-owned warehouses at the municipal level in each department. Parent-teacher committees are in charge of picking up the food from these delivery points, taking it to the schools, and storing and managing it for daily distribution.

Community committees are responsible for cooking and distributing the food to the children daily. The committees can choose whether to hire cooks, pay community members, or volunteer. A baseline survey done in early 2009 indicates that about 70 percent of the schools that were visited depend on volunteers to cook the food. These are generally women, mothers of children in the school. In about 30 percent of the cases, the committees hire cooks.

As a result of extensive training and sensitization over the life of the program, community participation and ownership is very high. The same baseline survey indicates that in almost 80 percent of the schools visited, parents participate in the cooking of the food, and in 70 percent of the schools they participate in the distribution of the food to the children.

Adequate infrastructure at the school level is a concern. About 67 percent of the schools have proper kitchen facilities. In the remaining 33 percent of schools, parents have to cook the food outside of school premises. The majority of schools do not have appropriate eating areas for children and almost 60 percent of schools lack potable water for cooking. These are some of the challenges that will be tackled in the coming years.

## How Did We Get Here? A Preliminary Study of the Transition Process of School Feeding in El Salvador

The transition to a nationally owned school feeding program in El Salvador took approximately 23 years to complete. This section reconstructs the chronology based on literature reviews and interviews with government and WFP staff.

The next part of this section identifies the different steps or actions that led to the current national program. The analysis of the transition process is done using the same five categories analyzed above: (1) policy framework, (2) institutional framework, (3) financial framework, (4) design and implementation, and (5) school-level arrangements and infrastructure. The analysis is designed to shed light on some of the key activities or triggers between the different stages of the transition.

### The Transition Process of School Feeding in El Salvador: Milestones

The transition to a nationally owned school feeding program in El Salvador took 23 years, as figure A1.1 illustrates. The program started in 1984 relying mainly on WFP for the funding and implementation (stage 1). In 1996, 12 years later, the program was inserted into a wider national school health program, Escuela Saludable, an initiative led by the country's First Lady. During this period, funds from donors (mainly the U.S. Agency for

**Figure A1.1    School Feeding Transition: Main Milestones of the Process in El Salvador**

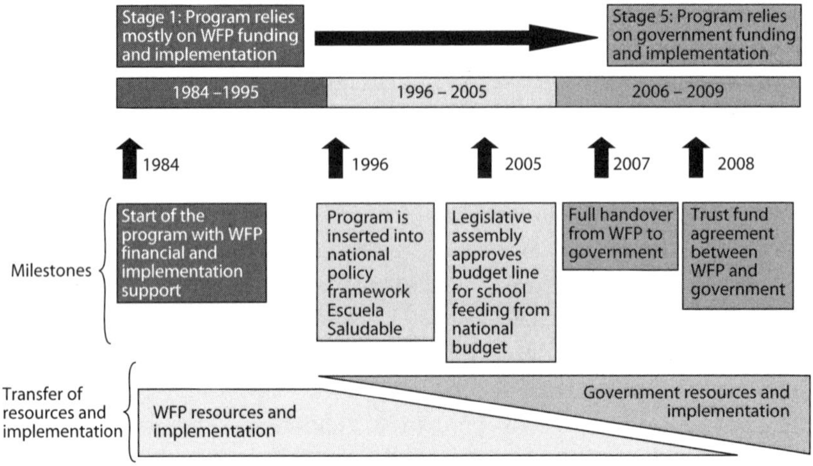

*Source:* Authors.

International Development) were secured to allow the government to start taking over designated portions of the program. In 2005, the Legislative Assembly approved a budget line for school feeding, institutionalizing the program within the national budget. The final handover of responsibilities from WFP to the government occurred at the end of 2007 (stage 5). Recently, the government requested WFP's support to manage the procurement and logistics of food commodities for the program using national funding under a trust fund (described in the previous section).

### The Transition Process
Figure A1.2 presents a schematic representation of the transition and the main actions that took place during the transition.

*Laying the foundations (1984–95).* During the first 11 years of implementation the program depended on WFP resources and capacity to operate. In that time, aside from food assistance, WFP also supported the Ministry of Education in building the institutional framework that would later support the program (including creating the program's technical and steering committee, and setting up a designated unit within the Ministry of Education). This process created the foundations that would later support the program within the Ministry of Education.

**Figure A1.2     School Feeding Transition: Steps of the Process in El Salvador**

| Stage 1: Program relies mostly on WFP funding and implementation | ⟶ | Stage 5: Program relies on government funding and implementation |
|---|---|---|
| 1984 – 1995 | 1996 – 2005 | 2006 – 2009 |

| Policy | Program starts at request of government under ministry | Program gets consolidated in the national policy framework | Program is considered one of the most important complementary programs |
|---|---|---|---|
| Institutional framework | Institutional framework for the program is established | Oversight and M&E are strengthened | Overall management capacity is strengthened |
| Funding | Funding for the program comes from WFP resources | Government seeks alternative funding | Program gets consolidated through a budget line from the national budget |
| Program design | Program starts with WFP food basket (rice, oil, meat, fortified drink) | Food basket, modalities, and targeting are changed and modified | Consolidation into one national food basket, expansion of coverage, and use of the program as a safety net platform |
| Community | Widespread training and sensitization for community and teachers | | |
| | Institutionalization of community participation by transitioning to school-based management | | |

*Source:* Authors.

*Institutionalizing the Program (1996–2005).* The period from 1996 to 2005 appears to be the critical period of transition. During this time, the government identified school feeding as a strategic program for the development of the country, inserted school feeding in the broader policy framework, explored sources of funding other than WFP, explored different modalities of implementation—including several changes in the food basket and in the delivery mechanisms—and increased its capacity to implement the program through extensive training. This period culminated with a stable source of funding for the program coming from the national budget, which effectively institutionalized the program and enhanced its sustainability considerably. This transition appears to have benefited from the leadership of high-level political champions, including two First Ladies and the current Minister of Education. Extensive capacity development was undertaken during this period.

*Learning by Doing and Looking Ahead (2006–08).* The ministry is increasingly confronted with several challenges of implementation related to the complete ownership of the program. According to government officials, the most challenging aspect of implementing the program has been the procurement and logistics arrangements, which are the two critical elements in service delivery for food-based programs. This new responsibility seems to have significantly burdened the ministry, especially in relation to its main responsibility related to education. The lack of experience in procurement, coupled with extremely high prices of food in the local market and changes in national legislation related to procurement, seem to have put the pipeline of the program in danger. In 2007 the ministry had planned to organize three food deliveries to the schools and could only deliver two, which left the schools without food during the last part of the year. As a consequence, the ministry requested WFP's assistance as a strategic partner for the program. Under the innovative arrangement, the ministry transfers resources to WFP under a trust fund for the procurement and delivery of food to the schools. WFP also provides technical assistance in the design and management of the program (see previous section).

### Preliminary Findings from the Process in El Salvador

The following sections present some of the key elements during that transition process, with the objective of deriving a set of critical factors that can be useful to other countries. It also analyzes some of the possible elements that the government might want to consider as it moves forward with the program in the coming years.

#### Findings on inserting the program in the policy framework

- The case of El Salvador illustrates that the transition to national ownership of school feeding takes time and a significant amount of planning and resources over the course of the transition stages. Indeed, it appears that the El Salvador experience has benefited from the explicit intention by the government and WFP to proactively manage the transition rather than just react to the situation.
- Awareness by the government that donor funding was declining as the country became a middle-income country precipitated the need to make a decision about the school feeding program beyond external assistance. Having a clear time frame for the duration of donor assistance gives the government time to manage the transition. The transition process in El Salvador benefited from a clear understanding among donors, implementing partners, and the government on the duration of external assistance and on the milestones in that process.
- In the case of El Salvador, the influence of high-level political champions (two First Ladies and now the Minister of Education) for school feeding has been decisive for the institutionalization of the program.

High-level support has translated into national financing and sustained political support for school feeding.

- The decision of making school feeding the cornerstone of the Escuela Saludable national flagship social program was based on sound information about the results and future potential benefits of school feeding in El Salvador. A strong knowledge base from data from the Ministry of Education and WFP served to inform the decision-making process at the policy level.
- Popular demand for the program has determined a great part of its success and its sustainability.

### Findings on strengthening the institutional framework of the program

- The capacity of the ministry to manage the program has increased over time with significant external support. The program started in 1984 with one government official assigned to school feeding. During the first decade the ministry created a dedicated unit to manage the program, with five officials and a director. In the early years the position of the director was funded by WFP. The current structure within the Ministry of Education has been strengthened significantly, with about 10 government officials dedicated exclusively to the program and a specific budget.
- The institutional framework was strengthened in a phased and highly planned manner. The ministry started by putting in place the decision-making and coordination structures (steering and technical committees), then establishing a specific unit within the ministry to manage the program, and finally strengthening individual capacities at various levels through training and sensitization. There was also considerable investment in technology with the establishment of a monitoring and evaluation system for the program, infrastructure, and supplies (such as motorcycles for field monitors). WFP provided the resources and technical expertise for most of these initiatives. At each stage, capacity development activities were carried out based on a baseline assessment of the situation and in-depth knowledge about the institutional gaps. Follow-up assessments were done to measure progress against predetermined capacity-development indicators.
- During the second stage of the transition, significant resources were invested in training and sensitization, including public officials in charge of the program at national, departmental, and local levels; and teachers, parents, and community members. The design and implementation of

this capacity-development effort was done with the participation of several units within the Ministry of Education. This also increased the level of ownership within the ministry. During the entire effort, some 80,000 parents and 10,000 teachers were trained. The entire effort was supported with resources from the Ministry of Education and WFP. It enhanced institutional ownership and quality of implementation and also involved the community in the program.

• Rotation of staff within the ministry and at the local level means that knowledge and capacity are weakened over time and there is a need for constant training and sensitization.

### Findings on financing the program

• The government has increased its capacity to finance the program over time, as figure A1.3 illustrates. School feeding direct costs depended exclusively on WFP resources from 1984 until 1999, and then slowly started to be financed by the government and donors until 2008, when it became exclusively financed by the government.

**Figure A1.3    Yearly Expenditure on School Feeding in El Salvador by Source of Funding, US$**

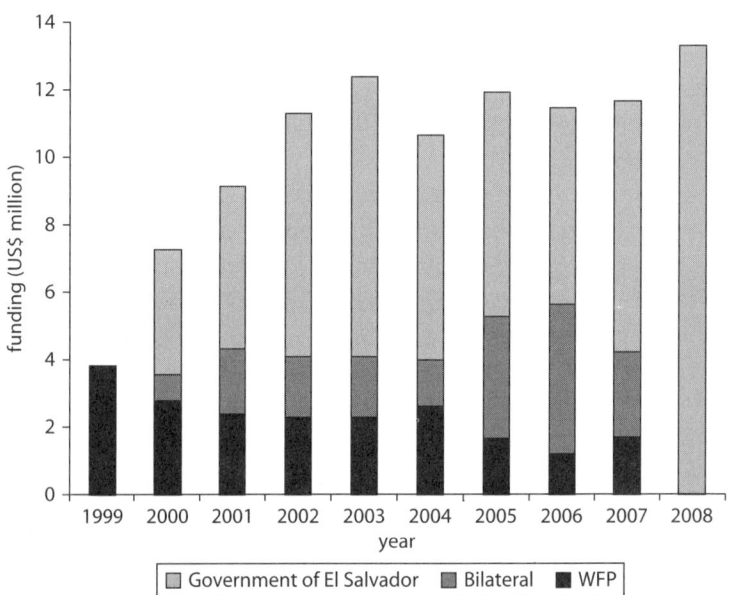

*Source:* Authors, using data from the Ministry of Education of El Salvador.

The Legislative Assembly approved a budget line for school feeding from national resources in 2005, marking an important milestone for the sustainability of the program.

- Figure A1.3 illustrates that the transition toward national ownership in El Salvador included a period of several years where the government found interim solutions for funding until national capacity was in place. One mechanism included using the proceeds of the privatization of the national telecommunications company to finance the program. This innovative solution was implemented thanks to a national law passed in 1999 that determined that the proceeds of the privatization would be put in a trust fund and that the interest gained would be allocated to social programs such as school feeding. To date, the trust fund has allocated about US$37 million to school feeding. In 2008, proceeds from the trust fund represented approximately 53 percent of the government's budget for the program.

- El Salvador was classified as a middle-income country during the second half of the 1990s, at which point donor assistance started to dwindle. In 1997, WFP decided to phase out its operation in El Salvador by 2003; a decision was postponed several times because of El Salvador's vulnerability to natural disasters, including Hurricane Mitch in the late 1990s. In response, the government started to look for alternative sources of funding among other donors, which resulted in U.S. Agency for International Development (USAID) and U.S. Department of Agriculture contributions for a number of years, and national sources of funding. Having a clear agreement with the government on the duration of donor resources facilitated the transition to government financing.

- A concrete handover strategy with WFP was put in place in 1997, with specific milestones. The government progressively took responsibility for the funding and implementation of the program.

- Future presidential elections in El Salvador will test the sustainability of the program. However, officials that were interviewed think that taking the program out of the national budget (which would mean reversing an act of the Legislative Assembly) would be very difficult and politically damaging.

### Main findings on the design of the program

- The case of El Salvador illustrates that it takes time to design an appropriate school feeding program, that there may be a need to revisit a program during the transition, and that there are several issues that need to be taken into consideration when designing an intervention. Changes in the design of the program in El Salvador were influenced by the different funding sources, the conditions in the country, the capacity of the government, the costs, and changes in policy. In recent years, the design of the program has been harmonized thanks to a more stable source of funding coming from national resources.

- The food basket was modified several times in the life of the program to reduce costs, accommodate new donor restrictions, and experiment with new modalities of service delivery. Three modalities can be discussed here:

  - *On-site meals* have been the predominant modality of the program since 1984. It has been implemented under the projects supported by WFP and USAID. The food basket, however, has changed over the years. WFP started providing rice, oil, canned meat, and a fortified drink. All of the commodities were internationally purchased except for the fortified drink. However, in 1996 WFP changed the food basket to include locally produced corn-soya blend instead of canned meat. This also brought the costs of the food basket down and allowed for a gradual government takeover of operations throughout the country.

  - *Fortified biscuits* were piloted with the help of WFP in early 1992. Although less expensive, the biscuits were very hard and dry, tasted a bit like iron, and were not well accepted by children. Evaluations showed that teachers, students, and parents were not satisfied with this new modality and attendance rates started declining. The ministry decided to discontinue the use of biscuits in late 1993.

  - *Direct transfer of resources to schools* was piloted by the government in 2001, which consisted of transferring the US$0.12 per child per day to schools. The director of the school was supposed to organize the purchase, cooking, and delivery of the food. This method was challenging because of lack of prior training and sensitization to the community, lack of capacity to monitor the program, and lack of previous planning. As a result, there was a significant reduction in the quality of the food, the modality overburdened the teachers, and there were some problems with accountability at the school level in some cases. This modality was eliminated in 2006.

- The food basket was standardized nationwide in 2007. The current modality is an on-site meal consisting of rice, beans, milk, sugar, and oil.

- The program was targeted initially by municipality following a WFP assessment in 1984. This meant that school feeding schools were scattered throughout the 14 departments in the country. A retargeting exercise supported by WFP in 1995 led to targeting by department (all the schools in a vulnerable department were targeted). This targeting exercise also served as a basis for government takeover of the program. WFP withdrew from all nonvulnerable districts and limited its operations to 7 of the 14 departments in the country, while the government took control of the remaining departments and schools.

- WFP has supported at least two national nutrition surveys and one targeting study that have served as the basis for the program. The ministry considers WFP's involvement in the process crucial because it has guaranteed the quality and impartiality of the process.

- As figure A1.4 illustrates, WFP's beneficiary caseload declined from 2000 until the full handover in 2008. The totality of beneficiaries of school feeding in El Salvador is now covered by the government. The absolute number of children has increased over the years. The program started reaching about 200,000 children in 1984 and now reaches more than 870,000 children. The program was expanded in 2008 to respond to the high food price crisis. Initially covering children in

**Figure A1.4    School Feeding Beneficiaries in El Salvador per Year by Implementing Agency**

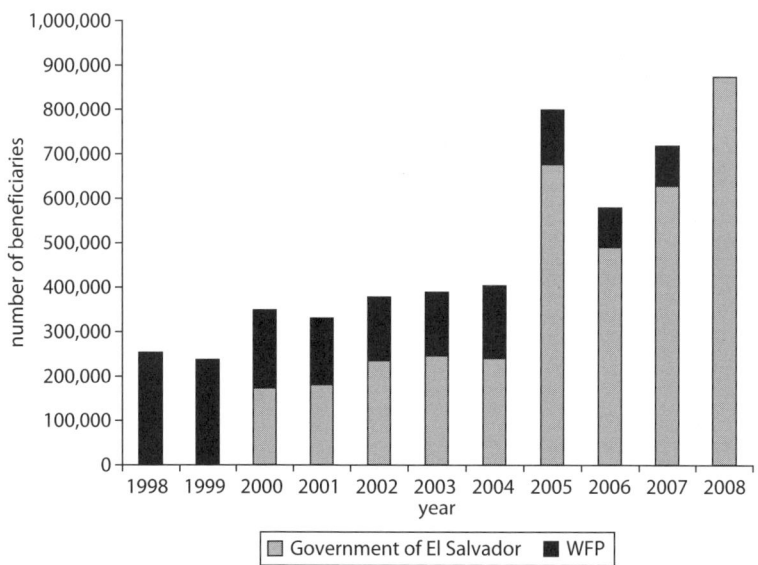

*Source:* Authors, using data from the Ministry of Education of El Salvador.

preprimary and primary education, it now covers lower-secondary students as well. Figure A1.4 illustrates changes in absolute coverage over the years by source of funding.

- The program reaches about 60 percent of the total number of children enrolled in basic education.

### *Main findings on implementation of the program*

- As with design, the implementation of the program has also changed during the life of the program. The transition from WFP to government implementation started in 1997. WFP withdrew from departments while the government took over schools that were previously supported by WFP. This allowed the government to slowly increase its capacity to manage the program with schools and communities that were already trained and sensitized.
- According to government officials, the transition of procurement and logistics was the last and most difficult part of the process, precisely because the government did not have the experience and had limited capacity to handle a large-scale procurement operation. Several government officials pointed to the fact that once the program was institutionalized and government owned after the 2005 Legislative Assembly decision, the Ministry of Education was faced with the challenge of actually implementing the program in all its complexity, a task that it was not prepared to take on. A consequence of this was the growing sense that the ministry was taking on functions that were not part of its core business and significantly hampered its ability to fulfill its main mandate to provide high-quality education to all children.
- A handover of implementation responsibilities does not necessarily mean that the government could not benefit from external assistance beyond the handover. Governments may benefit from external support even after a complete handover has taken place. In this sense, handover may not necessarily mean complete phase out from external assistance.

## Preliminary Conclusions

- The case study of El Salvador illustrates that the transition to national ownership of school feeding takes time and a significant amount of planning and resources over the course of the transition stages. Indeed, it appears that the El Salvador experience has benefited from the explicit intention by the government and WFP to proactively manage the transition rather than proceeding reactively. Some key actions in managing the transition include the following:

- Ensuring that there is a clear agreement between the government and partners on the duration of donor assistance and the milestones of a transition process.
- Allocating a significant amount of resources for capacity development at all levels. In El Salvador support appears to have been effective because it was planned based on an initial capacity assessment and monitored throughout. In-depth knowledge of the institutions and clear agreements with partners are also important.
- Finding interim financing solutions until national capacity to finance the program is in place. The capacity to finance school feeding, as with the capacity to implement the program, gradually increased during the transition. Interim financing was sourced from new donors and from other national sources.
- Institutionalizing school feeding within the national budget. There is a need to secure funds from the national budget in the long run for these programs. The process in El Salvador benefited from the support of high-level political champions for school feeding.
- Continuously revisiting the design of the program to enhance effectiveness and efficiency. The case of El Salvador illustrates that it might take time to get things right. Multiple modifications to the food basket, targeting mechanisms, and delivery modalities were needed.

• The transition to national ownership in El Salvador happened in phases, each characterized by specific strategic actions. There are some preliminary conclusions from El Salvador identifying the triggers or priority actions that facilitated the transition:

- One important first step in the transition from an externally supported program to one that is nationally owned is to set up the appropriate management structures within the institution designated to manage the program, in this case, the Ministry of Education. This includes creating a specific unit or division within the ministry, with appropriate levels of staff to manage the program.
- The second step is to integrate school feeding within the broader national policy framework. In this regard, a pre-established unit within the ministry, which has adequate information about the benefits of school feeding, is necessary to adequately position school feeding within the wider education and social protection sectors.

- ■ Once the two previous steps are in place, a period of intense change needs to be carefully managed. This includes finding alternative funding sources, revisiting the design of the program, and investing significantly in capacity development at all levels. This step may benefit from having the right information on the costs, the trade-offs, and the challenges of several aspects of design. Attention also could be paid to putting in place a comprehensive information management system for school feeding to assist in program implementation.
- Governments may benefit from external support even after a complete handover has taken place. In the case of El Salvador, the program is benefiting from technical assistance. In this sense, transition may not necessarily mean complete phaseout from external assistance.
- The five critical sustainability elements for school feeding in El Salvador are (1) a clear national policy framework, (2) a strong institutional framework, (3) national financing capacity, (4) sound program design and efficient implementation, and (5) community participation and local-level arrangements.

# Vulnerability Analysis and Mapping

## What Is VAM?

Vulnerability Analysis and Mapping (VAM) is a WFP information tool for beneficiary and geographical targeting. It provides information about who are the hungry poor and where they live. As an analytical tool, it also examines the causes of hunger and tries to answer a fundamental question for WFP: what is the most appropriate response in reducing vulnerability to food insecurity? Finally, as a program support tool, it provides decision makers with food security and vulnerability information for appropriate program design and targeting.

VAM efforts are guided by the following fundamental questions:

- Who are the food insecure and hungry?
- Where do they live?
- How many are they?
- Why are they vulnerable to food insecurity and hunger?
- How is their situation likely to evolve and what are the risks threatening them?
- What should be done to reduce their vulnerability to food insecurity?

VAM helps to strengthen the knowledge base on issues related to food security and vulnerability, improve targeting of food assistance, and facilitate partnerships with national governments in their efforts to establish and manage national food-assistance programs. To provide effective support in these areas, WFP is working on the design and implementation of food security monitoring systems—a regular update and outlook of the food security and livelihood situation of vulnerable populations—and has developed a Web-based information system (VAM Spatial Information Environment) to enable WFP to share VAM information with partners and donors.

## Overview of VAM Activities

VAM studies or activities, at minimum, seek to analyze data and information on the following themes:

- The broader context and environment
- Food availability
- Food access
- Food utilization
- Risks and vulnerability associated with these themes.

Maps are used for representing findings of analyses.
    VAM activities include

- A literature review
- Secondary data analysis
- Primary data collection with specific caveats to account for local contexts.

The outputs of VAM efforts—using the findings from data collection and analyses—are three types of products: analytical and assessment reports, food security monitoring systems, and the VAM Spatial Information Environment.

## Types of VAM Food Security Analyses and Assessments

WFP has several assessment tools to provide the right information at the different points of the program cycle.

- A Comprehensive Food Security and Vulnerability Analysis (CFSVA), also referred to as a precrisis baseline study, provides an in-depth picture of the food security situation during a noncrisis year (at normal times). A CFSVA contains a breadth of information (food consumption patterns, education, nutrition, markets, livelihoods); profiles of the food insecure; and an analysis of risks, vulnerability, and their underlying causes. It usually covers an entire country and is valid for up to five years.

The baseline study provides information to design recovery operations and country programs. It is used as a benchmark against which to measure change after a crisis. It informs contingency planning and preparedness.

- An Emergency Food Security Assessment (EFSA) is undertaken following a disaster or a shock. It covers geographic areas affected to determine the impact on households and their livelihoods and to provide response recommendations on food and nonfood assistance options. It is the basis for the design of relief and recovery operations. It identifies the number of people in need and the appropriate type and duration of assistance.

    The EFSA can be in the form of an initial, rapid, or in-depth assessment.

- Joint Assessment Missions (JAMs) are conducted in collaboration with the UN High Commissioner for Refugees to understand the situation, needs, risks, capacities, and vulnerabilities of refugees or internally displaced people (and host populations) with regard to food and nutritional needs.

- Crop and Food Supply Missions (CSAMs) are conducted jointly with the Food and Agriculture Organization, usually for emergencies related to agricultural production or overall food availability problems. The missions analyze the supply and demand for staple foods, estimate any uncovered staple food import requirement for the coming year, and analyze households' access to food.

- A Food Security Monitoring System (FSMS) is an ongoing activity to track changes in food security conditions. In particular, it provides advance notice of a deteriorating situation. It triggers an EFSA when the situation deteriorates progressively, or in case of a shock. It provides information to adjust contingency plans if the food security situation has deteriorated significantly and supports program monitoring by providing food security information about areas with and without assistance.

The various data collection activities (CFSVA, EFSA, FSMS) are aligned in their selection of indicators, timing, and methodology to enable the information from one assessment activity to feed into another, influence programming decisions at the most critical time, and enable solid monitoring and evaluation.

## Spatial Analysis and Mapping

WFP uses advanced technologies including Geographical Information Systems (GIS), innovative satellite applications, and Personal Digital Assistants to collect, manage, and analyze data. For example, by analyzing trends in rainfall patterns and regeneration of vegetation cover, potential biophysical threats to food security can be identified and monitored over time. WFP uses GIS to combine numerical household-level data with geographic factors to identify the root causes of food insecurity and vulnerability.

More information on WFP's food security analyses, guidelines, and assessment reports can be found at http://www.wfp.org/food-security.

# Setting Up School Feeding Programs

## Objective of the Tool

As the analysis in this document suggests, several elements critical to the sustainability of a school feeding program should be planned for at the outset. There are also trade-offs in the design that need to be addressed. This tool takes those elements into consideration with the objective of providing a checklist of the type of information, minimum conditions, and steps that are needed to set up a new school feeding program.

## Description of the Tool

This tool presents a series of steps or activities that may be followed when planning a new school feeding program. The checklist starts by detailing the information that will be needed to do a thorough analysis of the situation, identifying the problems and the context to determine whether school feeding is the appropriate intervention. After defining the objectives of the program, the tool provides guidance on the targeting mechanisms, rations composition, management and implementation structure, and school-level arrangements. The tool also includes guidance on how to plan for sustainability when designing school feeding programs.

## Step-by-Step Guide for Design and Implementation of School Feeding

| | |
|---|---|
| *Cross-cutting issues* | *To ensure quality school feeding programs that are sustainable and in line with international standards, the following issues need to be considered at each step of program design and implementation.* |
| Supporting government policies and building government capacity | School feeding programs should be owned by national governments and support government priorities, policies, and needs. Partnerships with national governments should be implemented in a manner consistent with the principles of ownership, alignment, harmonization, management for results, and mutual accountability. |
| Coordination and cooperation | Partnerships are central to delivering a school feeding package to children. Food inputs need to be combined with other resources to enhance education, health, nutrition, and equity outcomes. The Focusing Resources on Effective School Health (FRESH) framework and the Essential Package recommend the integration of school health and nutrition interventions. Programs must therefore be planned and implemented jointly with appropriate partners. |
| Community participation | While not overburdening families or communities, their commitment, participation, and contributions strengthen the implementation of school feeding programs and open up community development opportunities. |
| Gender | In cases where there are significant gender gaps in access to and completion of basic education, programs should include specific activities to address these imbalances. Implementation modalities should also be gender sensitive. |

## Formulating school feeding activities

| Step or activity | Key issues |
|---|---|
| Problem analysis | Carry out an assessment, in collaboration with the government, key partners, and local communities, to examine |

- Is there a need for school feeding?
- What problems should it address?
- Is it feasible?
- Is it in line with government priorities and policies?

The problem analysis considers the following main factors:

- *Prevailing situation in the country or region.* Onset or protracted crisis, post-conflict situation, postdisaster, or stable.
- *Need for school feeding.* Type and extent of problems regarding safety net (food security and income at household level; calorie intake at household and student level), education (access, retention, completion, learning, broken down by gender, regions, sociocultural groups; quality of education), nutrition (malnutrition rates including micronutrient deficiencies), and causes of these problems. Is there a need for school feeding?
- *Feasibility of school feeding.* Government institutional structures and implementation capacities; implementation capacities at school level; government financial capacity for school feeding; existence of complementary programs in, for example, school health and girls' education programs.
- *Government policies related to school feeding.* National policies, priorities, targets in school feeding, education, nutrition, social protection, and so on; does the proposed program fit into this context?

| | |
|---|---|
| **Objectives** | Clearly identify the program objectives and the expected outcomes, based on assessment results, corresponding to the country's specific context and to national policies. |
| **Targeting** | Identify relevant target groups and target areas, based on assessment results. Identify targeting mechanism.<br>This should consider: |

This should consider:

- Target areas (geographical areas with greatest need; accessibility, security of areas; availability of partner programs in areas; and so forth)
- Target groups (schoolchildren—all, specific groups such as girls; families and community members—all, families of schoolchildren, other specific groups)
- Types of schools to be assisted (educational level, public or private)
- Minimum criteria that schools have to meet for inclusion in the program (infrastructure, parents' committee ready to support school feeding, accessibility and security, and so forth).

Targeting criteria need to be clearly communicated and agreed on by all stakeholders.

Targeting criteria need to be respected during program implementation.

**Rations composition and food distribution modality**

Select type and composition of food rations in line with program objectives and practical aspects:

- Decide on appropriate modality (meals, snacks, take-home rations)
- Decide on frequency of distribution (daily, monthly, or other)
- Define culturally acceptable, nutritionally balanced food rations (type, quantity of commodities), taking into account

- Age range of target group
- Organization of school sessions
- Micronutrient needs of target group
- Energy needs
- Local food preferences
- Foods available locally
- Cost-effectiveness
- Infrastructure, fuel, and water availability
- Ease of preparation.

**Management structure**   Identify the government institution mandated with the implementation of school feeding at central, regional, and local levels (typically, Ministry of Education) and the management structure.

Identify capacity of this institution (staff, skills, funding, and so forth) and possible capacity-building activities.

Establish how the management of school feeding relates to the other responsibilities of the institution.

Identify existing planning and accountability structures in which school feeding will be included (technical working groups, steering committees, and so forth).

Establish the responsibilities of the central, regional, district, and school-level staff in the management of the program. Define roles, responsibilities of WFP and other partners in program management.

Sign letters of understanding between the government and each of the partners. Define arrangements for regular school monitoring and backstopping.

This may concern:

- Check on proper food storage, preparation
- Check records, reporting

- Check if basic school sanitation standards are met
- Check if program functions regularly, correctly
- Check on correct timing of food distribution (for example, serve food early to correctly address short-term hunger).

Define food procurement arrangements, taking into account:

- Local procurement whenever possible
- Cost-effectiveness
- Regularity of food supplies.

Define logistics system, including

- Food transport system
- Warehousing network
- Food transport to end point (school).

**School-level management**

Ensure necessary school infrastructure is available for school feeding implementation (storage, kitchen, water supply, cooking and eating utensils, and so forth).

If necessary, identify measures and partnerships to ensure that adequate infrastructure is developed.

Identify role of parents and local communities in school feeding implementation.

This can include:

- Provision of fuel wood, water
- Building storage, kitchen area
- Cooking, distribution of food
- Assistance with food transport, off-loading
- Participation in program monitoring and evaluation.

However,

- Make communities true program partners; don't limit participation to funding.
- Avoid overburdening communities and parents (risk to increase education costs to households).

|                                        |                                                                                                                                                                                                                                           |
| -------------------------------------- | ----------------------------------------------------------------------------------------------------------------------------------------------------------------------------------------------------------------------------------------- |
|                                        | • Avoid overburdening women (for example, as cooks)—women should be equal participants in the program.<br>• Plan for necessary training and community mobilization.                                                                        |
| **Monitoring and evaluation**          | Define system to monitor program functioning and results.<br>This includes examining the following:<br>• What information to collect (input, output, process, outcome indicators)<br>• How often to collect what type of information<br>• How to collect it<br>• How to use it<br>• Who should use it.<br>As much as possible, monitoring and evaluation indicators and methods should be aligned with national education management information systems (EMIS) or other sectoral information systems. |
| **Coordination and partnerships to maximize results** | Identify appropriate complementary activities to school feeding (in line with program objectives, expected outcomes), particularly for micronutrients and deworming.<br>Identify available partnerships, ways to implement such activities in targeted schools.<br>Set up intersectoral coordination mechanism, led by the government lead institution, and involving all school feeding stakeholders and partners. |
| **Planning for sustainability**        | Ascertain that the government is supportive of school feeding.<br>Main indicators include:<br>• The identification of school feeding in national poverty reduction strategies (as an education, social protection, nutrition policy)        |

- The inclusion of school feeding in sectoral plans, strategies, budgets
- A specific policy related to school feeding or school health and nutrition that specifies the objectives, rationale, scope, design, management structure, and funding of the program
- Commitment and plans to develop such a policy if not yet existing and to integrate school feeding in sectoral plans
- Contributions to the proposed school feeding program, within the countries' means
- A specific request for external assistance to school feeding (if appropriate).

Do not start or scale up a school feeding program without clearly stated government interest and support.

If necessary, provide technical support to help the government identify its position regarding school feeding.

Assess national capacity regarding school feeding policy development, planning, implementation, and funding.

- Identify capacity gaps that need to be filled by external assistance.
- Identify activities to gradually build national school feeding capacity and ownership.
- Define an agreed-on strategy (or a plan to elaborate one) with clear targets and milestones regarding increasing government financial and managerial responsibility for school feeding and related reduction and phasing out of external assistance.

Design program in way that lends itself to government takeover.

This concerns, for example:
- Food rations (use locally available, acceptable foods; do not create food habits and preferences difficult to sustain)
- Role of parents and local communities (payments for local services such as cooks may be difficult to sustain)
- Monitoring and evaluation (system to be aligned to national EMIS).

**Risk management, contingency planning**

Identify possible risks to program implementation (changes in resources, breaks in pipeline, change in country situation) and a strategy to contain and address them.

**Costing, budgeting**

Identify cost components for the program (one-off, continuing), such as:
- Start-up or scaling up costs (training, infrastructure, equipment, and so forth)
- Commodity costs
- Food transport, storage, handling costs
- Staff costs
- Management costs
- Costs arising at local level, to communities
- Cost of possible policy support, capacity-development activities.

Calculate costs for identified program period.

Identify possible funding sources (cash, in-kind), for example:
- Government
- WFP, other donors and partners
- Private sector
- Local communities.

# Revisiting School Feeding Programs

## Objectives of the Tool

The overall objective of this tool is to provide a framework to systematically assess the quality and potential for sustainability of school feeding programs. It introduces a new standard of good practice for quality and sustainability and introduces new benchmarks for current school feeding programs.

The specific objectives of the tool are to:

1. Provide a framework to assess school feeding programs and identify the factors that enhance or decrease their quality
2. Allow the identification of areas that require further attention from the government and stakeholders
3. Guide the design of strategies to tackle specific gaps
4. Provide baseline information that can be used to measure progress toward sustainability goals and serve as the basis for transition strategies
5. Facilitate dialogue between implementing partners and the government.

## Description of the Tool

This tool is meant to be used in a participatory and government-led exercise. Ideally, it is an interdisciplinary exercise involving policy, program, and procurement experts, among others. It is designed to guide in-country, multistakeholder discussions on school feeding and is divided into two main parts, a problem and status analysis and a sustainability assessment. The tool has been used as part of assessments to guide the redesign of existing school feeding programs; to provide a framework for national consultations and workshops among the government and stakeholders; and as a framework for case studies and evaluation exercises. One-, two-, or three-day workshop materials have been produced for this purpose.

The first part addresses the question of where the program is now and comprises a brief analysis of the context, including general poverty, hunger, education, and nutrition statistics, as well as an analysis of the current status of the school feeding program, including coverage, costs, and results. The second part is the main part of the tool and addresses the question of where the program is looking to go. This sustainability assessment is composed of a set of targets and guiding questions to assess the sustainability of the program. The analysis leads to a set of main findings corresponding to each target.

## The Tool—Part 1: Where Are We Now? Problem and Status Analysis

### Problem Analysis

This brief problem analysis is meant to give a general picture of the context but does not replace the detailed analytical exercise used to design a new school feeding program or to decide whether it is an appropriate intervention. This analysis is not exhaustive and should be geared toward capturing the main problems or issues that are relevant to school feeding from existing documents or analyses.

Guiding questions:

- What is the overall ranking of the country in measures of poverty and human development? How is the country doing in progress toward meeting Millennium Development Goal (MDG) 1?
- Are there specific factors that make the country more or less vulnerable (conflict, postconflict, natural disasters, and so forth)?
- Has the country been affected by the food, fuel, or financial crises? If so, in what way has this affected the most vulnerable? How are households coping with the crisis? Is the government taking any measures to respond to the crisis (that is, through social protection programs)?
- What are the main problems of the education sector, particularly primary education? They may be related to increasing enrollment,

narrowing the gender gap, improving completion rates, enhancing the quality of education, and the like. Are there any regional, gender, or socioeconomic differences? How is the country doing in progress toward meeting MDGs 2 and 3?

- Is there a high prevalence of micronutrient deficiencies or parasite infections among schoolchildren?
- Are there factors that increase children's vulnerability (orphan status, child labor, HIV status, and so forth)?
- What are the main problems of the agriculture sector? They may be related to agricultural production, lack of access to markets, poor postharvest practices, lack of functioning markets, and the like.
- What are the main food crops produced in the country and which regions are the most productive? What is the food processing capacity in the country (especially for fortified foodstuffs that could be used in school feeding)? Are there functioning markets and where are they located?

### Status of School Feeding

The aim of this section is to gain an overall understanding of the experience with school feeding to date, the coverage of the program, and its costs. The indicators below should be completed during the assessment.

- *General information on existing school feeding program(s).* Types of school feeding programs in the country and implementing partners. Objectives of the program, coverage of the program (absolute numbers and percentage of total school-age children in country), modalities of food delivered (on-site, take-home, snacks), cost of the program per child per year, funding sources for the current program.
- *Current food basket and nutritional standards.* Type of commodities provided, nutritional value of current rations, procurement arrangements for current rations.
- *Targeting.* Targeting criteria, geographical location of targeted schools (food-secure or food-insecure areas).
- *Current institutional arrangements.* Implementing partners, roles and responsibilities, capacities and challenges of implementing the program (especially from the government's side).
- *Current procurement arrangements.* Identification and description of any existing local production and local procurement arrangement for school feeding.
- *Lessons learned and challenges of current programs.* Analysis of evaluation documents or appraisal documents if available.

The following indicators should be collected:

- Education sector budget (in US$ and in percentage of the national budget)
- Primary education budget (in US$ and in percentage of the education sector budget)
- Primary education budget per child per year
- Cost of school feeding per child per year
- Number of children and number of schools covered under school feeding program
- Coverage of school feeding program, expressed as number of targeted children relative to the total number of primary schoolchildren, or the number of schools targeted relative to the total number of schools.
- Percentage of government contribution to the school feeding program.

## The Tool—Part 2: Where Do We Want to Go?

### Setting the Standards

In general terms, a quality school feeding program has the following in place: (1) a national policy framework, (2) sufficient institutional capacity for implementation and coordination, (3) stable funding, (4) sound design and implementation, and (5) community participation. Each of these quality standards is described below.

***National policy frameworks.*** The degree to which school feeding is articulated in national policy frameworks varies from country to country, but in general, a policy basis for the program helps strengthen its potential for sustainability and the quality of implementation. In all the cases where countries are implementing their own national programs, school feeding is included in national policy frameworks. Indeed, the largest programs have the highest level of politicization, for example, in India where the program is supported by a Supreme Court ruling and in Brazil where it is included in the Constitution.

In many developing countries, school feeding is mentioned in the countries' poverty reduction strategies, often linked to the education, nutrition, or social protection sectors, or in sectoral policies or plans. National planning for school feeding should ensure that the government has identified the most appropriate role for school feeding in its development agenda. With donor harmonization efforts underway, it is increasingly important that, if made a priority, school feeding is included in sector plans, which form the basis for basket funding or sectorwide approaches that determine the allocation of donor resources.

*Institutional framework and coordination.* The implementation of a school feeding program is generally the responsibility of a specific government institution or ministry. Best practice suggests that school feeding programs are better implemented if there is an institution that is mandated and accountable for the implementation of such a program. It also has to have adequate resources, managerial skills, staff, knowledge, and technology at the central and subnational levels to correctly implement the program.

*Stable funding and planning.* Governments plan and budget for their priorities typically on an annual basis based on a national planning process. With a general move toward decentralization, the planning process starts with village-level priority setting, which gets translated into local government (district) development plans. These plans form the basis for budgeting at the national level, making sure there is compliance with the national poverty reduction strategy and sectoral plans. The degree to which school feeding is included in this planning and budgeting process will determine whether the program gets resources from the national budget and whether it benefits from general budget support allocations.

In most countries supported by WFP, funding for the program comes from food assistance channeled through WFP and from government in-kind or cash contributions. As the program becomes a national program, it needs to have a stable funding source independent of WFP. This may be through government core resources or through development funding (sectorwide approaches, basket funds, Fast Track Initiative funding). Stable funding is a prerequisite for sustainability.

*Sound design and implementation.* School feeding programs should be designed based on a correct assessment of the situation in a particular country. It is important that the program clearly identify the problems, the objectives, and the expected outcomes in a manner that corresponds to the country's specific context. It is also important that the program target the right beneficiaries and choose the right modalities of food delivery and a food basket of the right quality. Complementary actions such as food fortification and deworming should be a standard part of any school feeding program.

School feeding requires a robust implementation arrangement that can procure and deliver large quantities of food to targeted schools, ensure the quality of the food, and manage resources in a transparent way. Countries and partners should carefully balance international, national, and local procurement of food to support local economies without jeopardizing the quality and stability of the food pipeline.

*Community participation and ownership.* School feeding programs that respond to community needs, are locally owned, and that incorporate some form of parental or community contribution, whether cash payment or in-kind, for example, through donated food or labor, tend to be the strongest programs and the ones most likely to make a successful transition from donor assistance. Programs that build this component in from the beginning and consistently maintain it have the most success.

### Assessing the Standards
The following section sets out targets for an effective and sustainable school feeding program and suggests some guiding questions to assess whether the targets are being met.

### *Standard: Sound policy framework*

1. **The national-level poverty reduction strategy or equivalent national strategy identifies school feeding as an education or social protection intervention, or both.**
   Guiding questions:

   - Does the country have a national-level poverty reduction strategy or similar policy or document?
   - Is school feeding mentioned in the poverty reduction strategy? If so, under which of the sectors is it mentioned? Are there targets to be achieved? Milestones set by the government?

2. **Sectoral policies and strategies identify school feeding as an education or social protection intervention (education sector plan, nutrition policy, social protection policy).**

   Guiding questions:

   - Is there an education sector plan? If yes, what are the main goals of the plan?

- Is school feeding mentioned in the education sector plan? What goals does it have? How specific is the education sector plan on school feeding? Does it have targets, time frames, and specifics on the implementation of the program?
- Is there any other macro-level policy that mentions school feeding? Examples may be the national nutrition policy, the social protection policy, or other standards and guidelines for education and training.
- If school feeding is mentioned in any of these, what are the objectives stated for school feeding? Do they differ from those in the poverty reduction strategy or in the education sector plan?

3. **There is a specific policy related to school feeding or school health and nutrition that specifies the objectives, rationale, scope, design, and funding of the program.**
   Guiding questions:

- Is there a school health and nutrition policy? If yes, does it mention school feeding? What are the objectives of the program under the policy? Does this policy state who is responsible for its implementation and the scope of the program?
- Is there a specific national school feeding policy? Do the objectives of school feeding correspond to those stated in the policy frameworks analyzed above? Does the policy specify the design of the program, targeted beneficiaries, scope, implementation requirements, and responsibilities and funding arrangements?

### Standard: Strong institutional structure and coordination

1. **There is a national institution mandated with the implementation of school feeding.**
   Guiding questions:

- Is there a specific ministry or institution with the mandate of managing and implementing school feeding?
- If it is not the Ministry of Education, does that institution have appropriate contact and communication with the Ministry of Education?

2. **There is a specific unit in charge of the overall management of school feeding within the lead institution at the central level and that unit has sufficient staff, resources, and knowledge.**

Guiding questions:

- Does the responsible unit in charge of implementing school feeding have a sufficient amount of staff? Are they working full time or part time on school feeding?
- Does the unit have enough resources to manage the program and to travel periodically on monitoring visits and the like?
- Is the unit's role proactive, in the sense that staff actively plan and make decisions for the program, or reactive in the sense that they mostly follow partners in planning for the program?
- How often does the unit meet with partners? Are meetings convened by the national implementation unit or by partners?
- Does the unit have staff that are trained and knowledgeable on school feeding issues?
- How is information about the program stored, analyzed, and managed? Is there a proper information management system in place for school feeding at the central level?
- How good is communication between the central and the local level for the implementation of the program? Does the unit in charge of implementation have direct information on the program or does it rely on external support?

3. **There is an operational intersectoral coordination mechanism in place that involves all stakeholders and partners of the institution.**
   Guiding questions:

- Is school feeding discussed in any national-level coordination body (technical working group, task force, or the like) that deals with school, health, agriculture, and nutrition issues, or quality issues, or special cross-cutting issues? If so, how often does this body meet? Do partners participate in this group?
- Does this group have a work plan or a regular list of tasks that it reports on? Is school feeding included in this work plan?
- Is there a national-level coordination body specifically for school feeding, led by the institution in charge of school feeding, that is operational and brings all stakeholders together regularly? Does it have a work plan or a set of targets or objectives?
- How often does it meet? Are meetings convened by the implementation unit or by partners?
- Is this coordination mechanism effective in making decisions for the program?

**4. There are adequate staff and resources for oversight at the regional level.**
Guiding questions:

- What is the responsibility of the regions related to school feeding?
- Do regional offices have sufficient staff and resources to fulfill their responsibilities?

**5. There are adequate staff and resources for design and implementation at the district level.**
Guiding questions:

- At the district or subnational level, who is involved in the implementation of the school feeding program? Are there specific staff assigned to the implementation of the program? What are their responsibilities and roles?
- Is there adequate infrastructure at the district level to perform the assigned tasks and responsibilities (computers, office space, cars, fuel, and so forth)?
- How is information about the program being captured at the district or subnational level? Is there an information management system in place at the district or subnational level?
- Do staff have sufficient skills and knowledge about the implementation of a school feeding program? What specific skills should be strengthened? Which ones could be further utilized?

**6. There are adequate staff, resources, and infrastructure for implementation at the school level.**
Guiding questions:

- Are there clear implementation arrangements at the school level? Do these rely mostly on the teachers or do they also include parents and the community?
- Are the people responsible for implementation trained on the management of the program (management and storage of food, entitlements, and reporting requirements)?
- Is there adequate storage capacity at the school level?

### Standard: Stable funding and planning

**1. School feeding is institutionalized within the national planning and budgeting process.**

Guiding questions:

- How do yearly priorities and resources within the government get decided and budgeted for? How does the national planning cycle work? Is school feeding included in the national planning process?
- How advanced is the decentralization process in the country? Do districts have the capacity to plan and budget their needs and request resources from the central level?
- If so, is school feeding included in district-level development plans? Do districts have a budget for school feeding?
- If the decentralization process goes down to the village level (where villages set their yearly priorities and plans), is school feeding included as one of the priorities at the village level?
- Overall, how embedded is school feeding in national- and local-level planning and budgeting processes?

2. **There is a budget line for school feeding and national funds from the government or from donors that cover the needs of the program.**
   Guiding questions:

- Does the government have provisions in the national budget to allocate resources to school feeding at the moment? If the government allocates resources, how much are they as a percentage of the total program requirement? What are these funds for (food, monitoring and evaluation, management, and so forth)?
- Is the government allocating a significant amount of resources to the program, or is it mostly funded by partners?
- Has the government progressively increased the amount of resources allocated to school feeding or has it been static in its contributions?
- Have there been conversations with partners on a possible government increase in financial responsibility?
- Is school feeding part of a sectorwide approach or a basket fund of the education, social protection, or agriculture sectors? Are there any donors financing the program through one of these mechanisms (for example, the World Bank)? If so, how much of the program is covered under these funding arrangements?
- Has the government received funds from the Education for All–Fast Track Initiative for school feeding?
- Overall, what is the capacity of the government to finance the program? Are there any potential donors that could be approached?
- How is the government planning to finance the program in the future?

*Standard: Sound design and implementation*

1. **The program has appropriate objectives corresponding to the context and the policy framework.**
Guiding questions:

- Are the objectives of the school feeding program coherent with the problem analysis? Are these objectives realistic taking into consideration the situation of the country?
- Do the objectives of the school feeding program match with the problem analysis and with the policy framework of the country? Are they the same as those stated in the poverty reduction strategy, in the education sector plan, and the social protection policy?

2. **Program design identifies appropriate target groups and targeting criteria corresponding to the objectives of the program and the context.**
Guiding questions:

- Are there explicit geographical targeting criteria and a proper targeting methodology that is consistent with the programs' objectives?
- Where are the schools located (food-secure or food-insecure areas)?

3. **Program has appropriate food modalities and food basket corresponding to the context, the objectives, the local habits and tastes, the availability of local food, and the nutritional content requirements (demand-side considerations).**
Guiding questions:

- Have the food modalities (on-site meals, snacks, take-home rations) been chosen based on the objectives of the program, the duration of the school day, and the feasibility of implementation?
- Are the commodities in the food basket locally or internationally purchased? Could more of the commodities be purchased locally?
- Are elements of the food basket not available in the country (for example, corn-soya blend in some countries)? If so, why were they chosen?
- What are foods currently produced in the country (and normally used by the population) that would be appropriate for school feeding? Are there locally processed foods or local businesses that might be able to supply food for the program?

- Could the food basket be modified to include more local food without sacrificing the nutritional content? Food basket should be compliant with national nutritional standards and food safety standards.
- How can local processing and fortification be included in the food supply chain? Is there capacity in the country?
- Would food basket modifications require extensive cooking or processing at the school or local level? Would this lead to environmental damage (fuel, fire wood, or the like)? Identify possible strategies to mitigate the environmental effects.
- What is the approximate demand of the school feeding program for local and regional foodstuffs (in total for the year, for the month, and per child per month)?

4. **Procurement and logistics arrangements are based on procuring as locally as possible, as often as possible, taking into account the costs, the capacities of implementing parties, the production capacity in the country, the quality of the food, and the stability of the pipeline (supply and procurement considerations).**
   Procuring as locally as possible depends on whether the program relies on in-kind or cash contributions, whether the elements in the food basket are available locally, and whether production and markets in the country are sufficient to guarantee the supply and the quality.
   Guiding questions:

- What are the main food crops and seasons, and where are the food-producing areas, including historic levels of production, and areas of regular food deficit?
- What are the major risks associated with crop failure (weather, economic shocks, and so forth) and existing risk mitigation mechanisms?
- If the school feeding program could be sourced locally, what type of risk management activities could be put in place to avoid jeopardizing the stability of the food pipeline?
- What are the main constraints in the country for agricultural productivity and how can these be tackled?
- Has there been an attempt at procuring more food locally? If so, what were the advantages, challenges, and constraints in procuring locally? Could these problems be solved by putting in place specific strategies to tackle them so that more food can be purchased locally?
- Have there been discussions with the government on possible procurement modalities for school feeding that can be more locally

appropriate, including the possibility of linking procurement with agriculture-related activities (that is, local-level support to small-scale farmers)?

- Has the Ministry of Agriculture been involved or contacted to make the connection between school feeding and national agricultural production? How can the agriculture sector be more involved in procurement for school feeding?
- Has the private sector been involved or could it be involved in making the connection between the farmers and market mechanisms (warehouses, associations, co-ops, and so forth)?
- At the local level, are the requirements for the school feeding program communicated to the agriculture sector so that more crops are grown for the program?
- What type of community structures, businesses, or efforts could be tapped into for processing or sourcing the food for the program?
- What would it take to buy the bulk of food requirements for the program? What type of systems or arrangements would be necessary to buy locally?
- Have there been any discussions on linking WFP's recent Purchase for Progress activities with the school feeding program? Purchase for Progress assessments could be used as the basis for school feeding procurement, or measures could be taken to support local markets, local processing capacity, or small-scale farmer associations.
- If the school feeding program could be sourced locally, how would the quality of the food be affected?
- If the school feeding program could be sourced locally, how would the costs of the program be affected?

5. **There is appropriate calibration of demand and supply, establishing what percentage of food demanded by the program can be sourced locally.**
   In developing home-grown school feeding programs, especially in the early stages, it is important to sustain and protect the existing food pipeline by maintaining current procurement practices (including food aid or purchases at the international, regional, or national levels), while beginning to test new procurement schemes that favor or support locally produced food. Thus, the bulk of the requirements of the school feeding program should still be sourced by traditional mechanisms, while a proportion of the current total demand of food for the program can be sourced locally. This is important to make sure the

program is not jeopardized, to allow time to learn and manage a complex activity such as procuring locally, and to avoid excessive market interferences that could generate problems for the program and for local capacity (small farmers, local businesses, and others). Local procurement can then progressively increase as the program evolves and mechanisms are put in place to guarantee the stability, nutritional content, and safety of the food.

Guiding questions:

- What percentage of the total food requirements of the program can be sourced from small-scale farmer associations, community groups, or local businesses?
- What percentage of the total food requirements can be sourced from food aid in-kind, or international or regional procurement?
- What type of procurement and supply interventions or initiatives will be started to test a more local approach?
- What are the main risks of shifting to locally produced food and how will they be mitigated during the initial stages?

6. **There is a functioning monitoring and evaluation system in place that forms part of the structure of the lead institution and is used for implementation and feedback.**
   Guiding questions:

- Is there a monitoring and evaluation plan for the school feeding program? Does the plan include data collection, analysis, reporting, feedback, indicators, guidelines, and tools?
- Who is involved in monitoring the program? Does the government at national and local levels have the capacity to monitor or does it rely on external support? Where do the periodic monitoring reports originate, at the government side and then get shared with external partners, or at the external partner side and then get shared with the government?
- Is the monitoring plan integrated into national education sector monitoring systems or information management systems and in subnational systems?
- Is there a budget for the monitoring and evaluation plan?
- Are there any problems monitoring outputs (food, nonfood items, and so forth)?
- Are there any problems monitoring outcomes (enrollment, attendance, and other measures)?

- How frequently are reports produced for the program?
- Is there a baseline for the program? Mid-term or end-of-term evaluation?
- How is information from the evaluations disseminated and translated into action or decisions?
- Is the information on the program reported at any national or local-level coordination mechanism (working group, task force, or other organization)?

### Standard: Strong community participation and ownership (parents, children)

1. **The community has been involved in the design of the program.**
   Guiding questions:

- Has the community been consulted in the design of the program?
- Has the community included school feeding as one of the priorities in village development plans?
- Are there any community-level structures that are used to establish communication (village councils, traditional authority structures, village elders, and the like)?
- Has the community been consulted on possible challenges to meeting the minimum requirements for school feeding and supported with strategies to overcome the challenges?
- Has the community been involved in deciding which products are provided in the food basket? If the community was more involved, would there be the possibility of mapping local-level businesses, processing capacity, and food production capacity to analyze the food basket of the program and the possibility of sourcing it locally?

2. **The community is involved in the implementation of the program.**
   Guiding questions:

- Is there a canteen or food management committee comprising representatives of parents, teachers, and students?
- Does this committee act as an interface between the community and the school, manage and monitor the school feeding program, and ensure good utilization of the food in the school?
- Do implementation arrangements avoid putting too much pressure and burden on teachers?
- Are community implementation arrangements efficient enough to not take up teaching or class time during school hours?

- Do implementation arrangements explicitly avoid involving children in the cooking or management of the food (especially girls)?

3. **The community contributes (to the extent possible) resources (cash, in-kind) to the program.**
   Guiding questions:

- Does the community contribute to pay the cooks or provide the firewood using in cooking?
- Does the community contribute food in-kind for the program to be given to children?
- Does the community contribute cash resources for the program?
- Overall, how significant is the community's contribution? Is it within households' means or is it burdening them excessively? What other contributions could they make that do not burden them?

# References

Abdul Latif Jameel Poverty Action Lab. 2005. "Education: Meeting the Millennium Development Goals." *Fighting Poverty: What Works* 1.

Adelman, S., H. Alderman, D. O. Gilligan, and J. Konde-Lule. 2008. "The Impact of Alternative Food for Education Programs on Child Nutrition in Northern Uganda." Draft, IFPRI, Washington, DC.

Adelman, S., H. Alderman, D. O. Gilligan, and K. Lehrer. 2008. "The Impact of Alternative Food for Education Programs on Learning Achievement and Cognitive Development in Northern Uganda." IFPRI, Washington, DC.

Adelman, S. W., D. O. Gilligan, and K. Lehrer. 2008. "How Effective Are Food for Education Programs? A Critical Assessment of the Evidence from Developing Countries." Food Policy Review No. 9, International Food Policy Research Institute, Washington, DC.

Ahmed, A. U. 2004. "Impact of Feeding Children in School: Evidence from Bangladesh." International Food Policy Research Institute, Washington, DC.

Ahmed, A. U., and C. del Ninno. 2002. "Food for Education Program in Bangladesh: An Evaluation of Its Impact on Educational Attainment and Food Security." Food Consumption and Nutrition Division, IFPRI, Washington, DC.

Ahmed, A. U., and M. Sharma. 2004. "Food-for-Education Programs with Locally Produced Food: Effects on Farmers and Consumers in Sub-Saharan Africa." International Food Policy Research Institute, Washington, DC.

Ahmed, T., R. Amir, F. Espejo, A. Gelli, and U. Meir. 2007. "Food for Education Improves Girls' Education: The Pakistan Girls' Education Programme." World Food Programme, Rome. http://www.schoolsandhealth.org/sites/ffe/Pages/KeyInformation.aspx.

Akshaya Patra Foundation. 2008. "School Lunch Program for Underserved Children in India." www.foodforeducation.org.

Alderman, H., D. O. Gilligan, and K. Lehrer. 2008. "The Impact of Alternative Food for Education Programs on School Participation and Education Attainment in Northern Uganda." Draft, World Bank, IFPRI, and University of British Columbia.

Alderman, H., and E. M. King. 1998. "Gender Differences in Parental Investment in Education." *Structural Change and Economic Dynamics* 9 (4): 453–68.

Andang'o, P. E. A., S. J. M. Osendarp, R. Ayah, C. E. West, D. L. Mwaniki, C. A. D. Wolf, R. Kraaijenhagen, F. J. Kok, and H. Verhoef. 2007. "Efficacy of Iron-Fortified Whole Maize Flour on Iron Status of Schoolchildren in Kenya: A Randomised Controlled Trial." *Lancet* 369 (9575): 1799–1806.

Belot, M., and J. James. 2009. "Healthy School Meals and Educational Outcomes." ISER Working Paper Series, Institute for Social & Economic Research, Essex, UK.

Bleakley, H. 2007. "Disease and Development: Evidence from Hookworm Eradication in the American South." *Quarterly Journal of Economics* 122 (1): 73–117.

Brinkman, H. J., N. Aberman, M. Baissas, D. Calef, C. Gingerich, L. Subran, A. Gelli, M. Sharma, and A. Stoppa. 2007. "Home-Grown School Feeding to Support Local Farmers in Africa." Paper presented to the World Food Programme "Home-Grown School Feeding Project Debriefing Meeting," Rome, July.

Brooker, S., P. J. Hotez, and D. A. P. Bundy. 2008. "Hookworm-Related Anaemia among Pregnant Women: A Systematic Review." *PLoS Neglected Tropical Diseases* 2 (9): e291.

Bundy, D. 2005. "School Health and Nutrition: Policy and Programs." *Food and Nutrition Bulletin* 26 (2 Suppl 2): S186–92.

Bundy, D., and B. Strickland. 2000. "School Feeding/Food for Education Stakeholders' Meeting." USAID Africa Bureau Office of Sustainable Development, Washington, DC. http://www.schoolsandhealth.org/pages/schoolfeeding.aspx.

Bundy, D. A. P., S. Shaeffer, M. Jukes, K. Beegle, A. Gillespie, L. Drake, S.-h. F. Lee, A.-M. Hoffman, J. Jones, A. Mitchell, C. Wright, D. Barcelona, B. Camara, C. Golmar, L. Savioli, T. Takeuchi, and M. Sembene. 2006. "School-Based Health and Nutrition Programs." In *Disease Control Priorities in Developing Countries: Second Edition*, ed. D. Jamison, J. G. Breman, A. R. Measham,

G. Alleyne, M. Claeson, D. Evans, P. Jha, A. Mills, and P. Musgrove, 1091–1108. New York: World Bank/Oxford University Press.

Caldes, N., and A. U. Ahmed. 2004. "Food for Education: A Review of Program Impacts." International Food Policy Research Institute, Washington, DC.

Ceesay, S. M., A. M. Prentice, T. J. Cole, F. Foord, E. M. E. Poskitt, L. T. Weaver, and R. G. Whitehead. 1997. "Effects on Birth Weight and Perinatal Mortality of Maternal Dietary Supplements in Rural Gambia: 5 Year Randomised Controlled Trial." *British Medical Journal* 315 (7111): 786–90.

Del Rosso, J. M. 1999. "School Feeding Programs: Improving Effectiveness and Increasing the Benefit to Education. A Guide for Program Managers." Partnership for Child Development, Oxford, UK.

Del Rosso, J. M., and T. Marek. 1996. *Class Action: Improving School Performance in the Developing World through Better Health and Nutrition.* Washington, DC: World Bank.

Devereux, S., R. Sabates-Wheeler, B. Guenther, A. Dorward, C. Poulton, and R. Al-Hassan. 2008. "Linking Social Protection and Support to Small Farmer Development." FAO, Rome.

Dréze, J., and G. Kingdon. 2001. "School Participation in Rural India." *Review of Development Economics* 5 (1): 1–24.

Edström, J., H. Lucas, R. Sabates-Wheeler, and B. Simwaka. 2008. "A Study of the Outcomes of Take-Home Food Rations for Orphans and Vulnerable Children in Communities Affected by AIDS in Malawi: A Research Report." UNICEF ESARO, Nairobi.

FAO (Food and Agriculture Organization of the United Nations). 2007. *The State of Food and Agriculture 2007.* Rome: FAO.

———. 2008. *The State of Food Insecurity in the World 2008.* Rome: FAO.

FAO, WHO, and UN University. 2004. "Human Energy Requirements: Report of a Joint FAO/WHO/UNU Expert Consultation." FAO Food and Nutrition Technical Report Series 1, Rome.

Fiszbein, A., N. Schady, F. H. G. Ferreira, M. Grosh, N. Kelleher, P. Olinto, and E. Skoufias. 2009. *Conditional Cash Transfers: Reducing Present and Future Poverty.* A World Bank Policy Research Report. Washington, DC: World Bank.

Frankenberg, E., K. Beegle, B. Sikoki, and D. Thomas. 1998. "Health, Family Planning, and Well-Being in Indonesia During an Economic Crisis." RAND, Santa Monica, CA.

Galasso, E., and M. Ravallion. 2005. "Decentralized Targeting of an Antipoverty Program." *Journal of Public Economics* 89 (4): 705–27.

Galloway, R., E. Kristjansson, A. Gelli, U. Meir, F. Espejo, and D. Bundy. Forthcoming. "School Feeding: Costs and Outcomes." *Food and Nutrition Bulletin.*

Gelli, A., N. Al-Shaiba, and F. Espejo. Forthcoming. "The Costs and Cost-Efficiency of Providing Food through Schools in Areas of High Food Insecurity." *Food and Nutrition Bulletin.*

Gelli, A., K. Izushi, Z. Islam, M. Matthew, and F. Espejo. 2006. "The Costs and Outcomes of Fortified Biscuit Interventions on Primary School-Age Children." World Food Programme, Rome.

Gelli, A., U. Meir, and F. Espejo. 2007. "Does Provision of Food in School Increase Girls' Enrollment? Evidence from Schools in Sub-Saharan Africa." *Food and Nutrition Bulletin* 28 (2): 149–55.

Grantham-McGregor, S. M., and C. Ani. 2001. "A Review of Studies on the Effect of Iron Deficiency on Cognitive Development in Children." *Journal of Nutrition* 131 (2): 649S–6S.

Grigorenko, E. L., R. J. Sternberg, M. Jukes, K. Alcock, J. Lambo, D. Ngorosho, C. Nokes, and D. A. Bundy. 2006. "Effects of Antiparasitic Treatment on Dynamically and Statically Tested Cognitive Skills over Time." *Journal of Applied Developmental Psychology* 27 (6): 499–526.

Grosh, M., C. del Ninno, and E. D. Tesliuc. 2008. "Guidance for Responses from the Human Development Sector to Rising Food and Fuel Prices." World Bank, Washington, DC.

Grosh, M., C. del Ninno, E. Tesliuc, and A. Ouerghi. 2008. *For Protection & Promotion: The Design and Implementation of Effective Safety Nets.* Washington, DC: World Bank.

Gulani, A., C. Nagpal, C. Osmond, and H. P. S. Sachdev. 2007. "Effect of Administration of Intestinal Anthelminthic Drugs on Haemoglobin: Systematic Review of Randomised Controlled Trials." *British Medical Journal* 334 (7603): 1095.

Hamdani, S. 2008. "Micronutrient Sprinkles to Address Multiple Deficiencies in School Age Children." WFP School Feeding, Rome.

Horton, S. 1992. "Unit Costs, Cost-Effectiveness and Financing of Nutrition Interventions." Policy Research Working Paper No. 952, World Bank, Washington, DC.

Jacoby, E., S. Cueto, and E. Pollitt. 1996. "Benefits of a School Breakfast Programme among Andean Children in Huaraz, Peru." *Food and Nutrition Bulletin* 17 (1): 54–64.

Jacoby, H. G. 2002. "Is There an Intrahousehold 'Flypaper Effect'? Evidence from a School Feeding Programme." *The Economic Journal* 112 (476): 196–221.

Jukes, M. C. H., L. J. Drake, and D. A. P. Bundy. 2008. *School Health, Nutrition and Education for All: Levelling the Playing Field.* Cambridge, MA: CABI Publishing.

Jukes, M. C. H., C. A. Nokes, K. J. Alcock, J. K. Lambo, C. Kihamia, N. Ngorosho, A. Mbise, W. Lorri, E. Yona, L. Mwanri, A. D. Baddeley, A. Hall, and D. A. P. Bundy. 2002. "Heavy Schistosomiasis Associated with Poor Short-Term Memory and Slower Reaction Times in Tanzanian School Children." *Tropical Medicine and International Health* 7 (2): 104–17.

Kattan, R. B. 2006. "Implementation of Free Basic Education Policy." Education Working Paper Series, World Bank, Washington, DC.

Kazianga, H., D. de Walque, and H. Alderman. 2009. "Educational and Health Impact of Two School Feeding Schemes: Evidence from a Randomized Trial in Rural Burkina Faso." Working Paper, World Bank, Washington, DC.

Kristjansson, E., V. Robinson, M. Petticrew, B. MacDonald, J. Krasevec, L. Janzen, T. Greenhalgh, G. Wells, J. MacGowan, A. Farmer, B. J. Shea, A. Mayhew, and P. Tugwell. 2007. "School Feeding for Improving the Physical and Psychosocial Health of Disadvantaged Elementary School Children." *Cochrane Database of Systematic Reviews* 1.

Lambers, W. 2008. "Interview: Abou Guindo of the UN World Food Programme in Mali." Ending World Hunger. *Blogcritics Magazine*.

Levinger, B. 1986. "School Feeding Programs in Developing Countries: An Analysis of Actual and Potential Impact." AID Evaluation Special Study No. 30, USAID, Washington, DC.

———. 1996. "Nutrition, Health and Education for All." Education Development Center and United Nations Development Programme, New York.

———. 2005. "School Feeding, School Reform, and Food Security: Connecting the Dots." *Food and Nutrition Bulletin* 26 (2 Suppl 2): S170–S178.

Lindert, K., E. Skoufias, and J. Shapiro. 2006. "How Effectively Do Public Transfers Redistribute Income in LAC?" In "Redistributing Income to the Poor and to the Rich: Public Transfers in Latin America and the Caribbean," ed. K. Lindert, E. Skoufias, and J. Shapiro, World Bank, Washington, DC.

Lukito, W., S. Muslimatun, U. Fahmida, D. H. Maskar, S. Fitriyanti, L. Seniati, M. Widjaja-Erhardt, D. O. Francisca, and L. N. Natasha. 2006. "Evaluation Survey: WFP Nutrition Rehabilitation Program through Primary School 2004–2006." WFP Indonesia and SEAMEO.

Mali Ministry of Basic Education. 2008. "National Policy for School Feeding in Mali." Bamako.

McKay, H., L. Sinisterra, A. McKay, H. Gomez, and P. Lloreda. 1978. "Improving Cognitive Ability in Chronically Deprived Children." *Science* 200 (4339): 270–8.

Miguel, E., and M. Kremer. 2004. "Worms: Identifying Impacts on Education and Health in the Presence of Treatment Externalities." *Econometrica* 72 (1): 159–217.

NEPAD (New Partnership for Africa's Development). 2007. "HGSF High-Level Consultation Ghana, Final Report of Proceedings." Ghana WFP Country Office.

Nokes, C., S. M. Grantham-McGregor, A. W. Sawyer, E. S. Cooper, B. A. Robinson, and D. A. Bundy. 1992. "Moderate to Heavy Infections of *Trichuris trichiura* Affect Cognitive Function in Jamaican School Children." *Parasitology* 104 (3): 539–47.

OECD (Organisation for Economic Co-operation and Development). 2006. "The Challenge of Capacity Development: Working Towards Good Practice." DAC Guidelines and Reference Series, Paris.

Powell, C. A., S. P. Walker, S. M. Chang, and S. M. Grantham-McGregor. 1998. "Nutrition and Education: A Randomized Trial of the Effects of Breakfast in Rural Primary School Children." *American Journal of Clinical Nutrition* 68: 873–9.

Ravallion, M., and Q. Wodon. 1998. "Evaluating a Targeted Social Program when Placement is Decentralized." Policy Research Working Paper, Development Research Group, World Bank, Washington, DC.

Schady, N. 2008. "The Impact of an Economic Contraction on Human Capital: Evidence from LAC and the World." Presentation at the World Bank, Washington, DC, May.

Semba, R. D., S. de Pee, K. Sun, M. Sari, N. Akhter, and M. W. Bloem. 2008. "Effect of Parental Formal Education on Risk of Child Stunting in Indonesia and Bangladesh: A Cross-Sectional Study." *Lancet* 371 (9609): 322–8.

Seshadri, S., and T. Gopaldas. 1989. "Impact of Iron Supplementation on Cognitive Functions in Preschool and School-Aged Children: The Indian Experience." *American Journal of Clinical Nutrition* 50 (3 Suppl): 675–84.

Simeon, D. T. 1998. "School Feeding in Jamaica: A Review of its Evaluation." *American Journal of Clinical Nutrition* 67 (4): 790s–4s.

Simeon, D. T., and S. Grantham McGregor. 1989. "Effects of Missing Breakfast on the Cognitive Functions of School Children of Differing Nutritional Status." *American Journal of Clinical Nutrition* 49 (4): 646–53.

Simeon, D. T., S. M. Grantham-McGregor, and M. S. Wong. 1995. "*Trichuris trichiura* Infection and Cognition in Children: Results of a Randomized Clinical Trial." *Parasitology* 110 (4): 457–64.

Soemantri, A. G., E. Pollitt, and I. Kim. 1985. "Iron Deficiency Anaemia and Educational Achievement." *American Journal of Clinical Nutrition* 42 (6): 1221–8.

Sonnino, R. 2007. "Local School Meals in East Ayrshire, Scotland: A Case Study." Paper presented to the World Food Programme.

Studdert, L. J., Soekirman, K. M. Rasmussen, and J.-P. Habicht. 2004. "Community-Based School Feeding during Indonesia's Economic Crisis:

Implementation, Benefits, and Sustainability." *Food and Nutrition Bulletin* 25 (2): 156–65.

Sudan Ministry of General Education. 2008. "Baseline Survey on Basic Education on the Northern States of Sudan." Directorate General of Educational Planning.

Svensson, M. 2009. "School Feeding: Realizing the Right to Education. A Legal Analysis." Draft, Master's Thesis for the University of Göteborg School of Law.

Tan, J.-P., J. Lane, and G. Lassibille. 1999. "Student Outcomes in Philippine Elementary Schools: An Evaluation of Four Experiments." *World Bank Economic Review* 13 (3): 493–502.

UNESCO. 2008. UNESCO Institute for Statistics. http://stats.uis.unesco.org.

van Stuijvenberg, M. E., J. D. Kvalsvig, M. Faber, M. Kruger, D. G. Kenoyer, and A. J. S. Benade. 1999. "Effect of Iron-, Iodine-, and Beta-Carotene-Fortified Biscuits on the Micronutrient Status of Primary School Children: A Randomized Controlled Trial." *American Journal of Clinical Nutrition* 69 (3): 497–503.

Vegas, E., and J. Petrow. 2007. *Raising Student Learning in Latin America: The Challenge for the 21st Century.* Latin American Development Forum Series. Washington, DC: World Bank.

Vermeersch, C., and M. Kremer. 2004. "Schools Meals, Educational Achievement and School Competition: Evidence from a Randomized Evaluation." Policy Research Working Paper No. 2523, World Bank, Washington, DC.

Watkins, W. E., and E. Pollitt. 1997. "'Stupidity or Worms': Do Intestinal Worms Impair Mental Performance?" *Psychological Bulletin* 121: 171–91.

WFP (World Food Programme). 2003. "Exit Strategies for School Feeding: WFP's Experience." WFP/EB.1/2003/4/C, WFP, Rome.

———. 2007a. "Checklist for the Use of Milk in School Feeding Programmes." Unpublished, School Feeding Service, Nutrition Service, WFP, Rome.

———. 2007b. "Standard Project Report: Cambodia Protracted Relief and Recovery Operation." SPR10305.1, World Food Programme, Rome.

———. 2007c. "Status of School Feeding in WFP Phase-Out Countries." WFP, Rome.

———. 2007d. "Summary Report of the Thematic Evaluation of School Feeding in Emergency Situations." WFP/EB.A/2007/7-A, WFP, Rome.

———. 2008a. "Purchase for Progress: Connecting Farmers to Markets." http://wfp.org/p4p/.

———. 2008b. "Summary Report of the Evaluation of WFP's Capacity Development Policy and Operations." Rome.

———. 2009. "Home-Grown School Feeding: A Framework for Action." WFP, Rome.

WFP and UNICEF. 2005. "The Essential Package: Twelve Interventions to Improve the Health and Nutrition of School-Age Children." WFP, Rome.

WFP Annual Performance Report. 2006a. "Capacity-building in Ecuador." World Food Programme, Rome.

————. 2006b. "Capacity-building in El Salvador." World Food Programme, Rome.

WFP Pakistan. 2005. "Situation Analysis: WFP's Assistance to Girl's Primary Education in Selected Districts of NWFP." WFP Pakistan, Islamabad.

Whaley, S. E., M. Sigman, C. Neumann, N. Bwibo, D. Guthrie, R. E. Weiss, S. Alber, and S. P. Murphy. 2003. "The Impact of Dietary Intervention on the Cognitive Development of Kenyan School Children." *Journal of Nutrition* 133 (11): 3965S–71S.

World Bank. 2000. "Panama Poverty Assessment: Priorities and Strategies for Poverty Reduction." World Bank, Washington, DC.

————. 2008. PovcalNet. http://go.worldbank.org/NT2A1XUWP0.

# Index

*Boxes, figures, and tables are indicated by b, f, and t, respectively.*

155

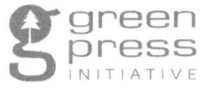